Pediatric Nutrition Handbook: An Algorithmic Approach

To the inspirations in my life,
Rebecca, Elias, and Sadie and the
foundation from which I grew,
Mom and Dad.

– David L. Suskind

A special acknowledgment to my children
Natalie and Charles, who taught me
to "relax" about childhood feeding and
appreciate every day of life!

– Polly Lenssen

Pediatric Nutrition Handbook
An Algorithmic Approach

Edited by

David L. Suskind, MD
Associate Professor of Pediatrics
University of Washington
Division of Gastroenterology, Hepatology and Nutrition
Seattle Children's Hospital

and

Polly Lenssen, MS, RD, CD, FADA
Director, Clinical Nutrition
Seattle Children's Hospital

WILEY-BLACKWELL

A John Wiley & Sons, Ltd., Publication

Library of Congress Cataloging-in-Publication Data

Pediatric nutrition handbook : an algorithmic approach / edited by David L. Suskind and Polly Lenssen.
    p.   ;   cm.
  Includes bibliographical references and index.
  ISBN-13: 978-0-4706-5995-3 (pbk. : alk. paper)
  ISBN-10: 0-470-65995-5 (pbk. : alk. paper)   1. Children–Nutrition–Handbooks, manuals, etc.
2. Nutrition disorders in children–Handbooks, manuals, etc.   I. Suskind, David L.   II. Lenssen, Polly.
  [DNLM: 1. Child Nutrition Disorders–Handbooks.   2. Adolescent.   3. Child.
4. Gastrointestinal Diseases–Handbooks.   5. Infant Nutrition Disorders–Handbooks.   6. Infant.
7. Metabolism, Inborn Errors–Handbooks. WS 39]
  RJ206.P3625   2011
  618.92–dc23

                                                                    2011020646

A catalogue record for this book is available from the British Library.

Set in 10 on 12.5 pt Sabon by Toppan Best-set Premedia Limited

Printed and bound in Malaysia by Vivar Printing Sdn Bhd

1   2011

Contents

Preface

Each year, millions of children throughout the world are subjected to the life-threatening ravages of malnutrition. The nutritional issues that children face today have radically changed as knowledge on disease processes as well as their treatments have improved.

We know the effect of nutrition is profound. Good nutrition not only assures proper growth and development, but it also enables each organ system to do its job properly. In ill children, nutrition is paramount, affecting both morbidity and mortality. As medicine has specialized, the nutritional care of children has also become increasingly specialized. This handbook serves as a broad guide to the nutritional care for the developing infant and child as well as for children with specialized medical needs.

This handbook is the fruition of a long-held dream by many at Seattle Children's Hospital to standardize the nutritional care of our patients. Collectively, it represents years of experience and specialized knowledge in the nutritional assessment and care of infants, children, and teens.

We would like to recognize our contributors for their time and effort. Additional thanks to the many reviewers who both recommended content and analyzed all the chapters. Our hope is that all health care providers – residents, nurses, dietitians, and other clinicians – find the handbook helpful. We welcome feedback to improve future publications.

David L. Suskind
Polly Lenssen

This handbook is designed to assist healthcare practitioners deal with the large number of nutritional issues which present during childhood. It is intended to be a quick reference only and not an in-depth review of either nutritional or medical issues that occur in childhood. This book is an educational resource only and none of its content is meant to be standard of care. The authors would like to acknowledge Seattle Children's Hospital for its commitment to nutrition and the importance it plays in a child's health.

Foreword

The idea that good nutrition is essential for the optimal development of a child and to the child's evolvement to a healthy adulthood seems simple. But translating that simple idea to effective truth is a challenge. It's for that reason that this book is so important. David L. Suskind, M.D,. and Ms. Polly Lenssen have created, with Seattle's most expert nutritionists, a book which is essential for every physician and health worker dealing with children. They have, for the first time in medical history, provided the pediatric health worker with a systematic algorithmic approach to the nutritional support of all children and, most importantly, children with primary and secondary nutritional deficiencies.

With rare comprehensiveness, this volume provides the mechanism for the nutritional assessment of infants and adolescents as well as a comprehensive list of the pediatric diseases that impact on the nutritional status of children including the cardiac, gastrointestinal, metabolic, neurologic, pulmonary, renal, and rheumatologic systems.

Dr. Suskind and Ms. Lenssen have described the important role played by nutrition in maintaining the cellular integrity of the body, demonstrating that, without this integrity, organs and systems fail and the nutritional complications of disease processes contribute to the morbidity and mortality associated with the underlying disease. By developing an inductive algorithmic approach to the handling of these nutritional problems they provide those responsible for pediatric care a systematic, logical, effective approach to dealing with the nutritional impact of disease.

Pediatric Nutrition Handbook: An Algorithmic Approach is an outstanding textbook, critical to good pediatric care. I personally want to congratulate the editors and all of the contributors. Their contribution to this book is invaluable.

Robert Suskind, M.D.
Former Founding/Regional Dean
Professor of Pediatrics/Director of International Health
Paul L. Foster School of Medicine
Texas Tech Health Science University at El Paso
El Paso, Texas

Acknowledgments

Much appreciation to Melissa Redding, for her astounding abilities, diligence, and dedication to this project, and Mi Ae Lipe, for her commitment, enthusiasm, and attention to detail. For the nutrition assessment chapters, we would like to acknowledge the contributions of the clinical nutrition staff over many years in developing our standard guidelines.

We would also like to thank the many reviewers whose help was essential:

Tyler Burpee, MD
Dennis Christie, MD
Ronald Dick, MD
Allison Eddy, MD
Patricia Fechner, MD
Joseph Flynn, MD
Ian Glass, MD, MB, ChB
Sidney Gospe, MD, PhD
Sihoun Hahn, MD, PhD
Coral Hanevold, MD
Doug Hawkins, MD
Simon Horslen, MB, ChB
Craig Jackson, MD, MHA
Mark Lewin, MD
Lenna Liu, MD, MPH

David Loren, MD
Lawrence Merritt, MD
Melissa Mortensen, MS, RD, CD, CSP
Kathryn Ness, MD, MS
Edward Novotny, MD
Aaron Owens, MS, RD, CD, CSP
Cate Pihoker, MD
Gregory Redding, MD
Russell Saneto, DO, PhD
Jordan Symons, MD
Joel S. Tieder, MD, MPH
Ghassan Wahbeh, MD
John Waldhausen, MD
Linda Wallen, MD
Jerry Zimmerman, MD

Contributors

Note: All the contributors are based at the Seattle Hospital for Children, Seattle, Washington.

Christine Avgeris, MS, RD, CD, CDE
Lee Bossung Sweeney, MN, RN, IBCLC
Susan Casey, RD, CD
Kim Cooperman, MS, RD, CD
Elaine Cumbie, MS, RD, CD, CDE
Cheryl Davis, RD, CD, CNSC
Alicia Dixon Docter, MS, RD, CD
Melissa Edwards, RD, CD
Matt Giefer, MD
Tran Hang, MS, RD, CD, CDE
Simon Horslen, MB, ChB
Kathy Hunt, RD, CD
Kim Kellogg, MS, RD, CD
Crystal Knight, MD
Polly Lenssen, MS, RD, CD, FADA
Marta Mazzanti, MS, RD, CD
Kelly McKean, MS, RD, CD
Heather Paves, MS, RD, CD
Maura Sandrock, MS, RD, CD
Claudia Sassano-Miguel
Peggy Solan, RD, CD
Jenny Stevens, RD, CD, CNSC
David L. Suskind, MD
Kirsten Thompson, RD, CD, MPH

Chapter 1
General Nutrition

1.1 General Pediatric Nutrition Assessment

Cheryl Davis and the Clinical Nutrition Department

The authors of the nutrition assessment chapters would like to acknowledge the contributions of the clinical nutrition staff over many years in developing standard guidelines.

1.1.1 Weight

1. **Weigh on digital or calibrated scale** (infant scale: 0–36 months; standing scale >3 years).
2. **Plot on age- and sex-appropriate World Health Organization (WHO) growth chart.**
3. **Weight-for-age:** A measure for acute malnutrition.
4. **Interpretation:** Gómez classification (Gómez et al., 1956).

First-degree malnutrition	76–90% of theoretical weight for age
Second-degree malnutrition	61–75% theoretical weight for age
Third-degree malnutrition	≤60% theoretical weight for age

1.1.2 Height or Length

1. **Recumbent length (up to 36 months):** Measure on length board with one person at the head and one at the feet, and plot on a 0–36-month sex-appropriate WHO growth chart. Do not use a tape measure.
2. **Stature (2–20 years):** Measure with a stadiometer and plot on a 2–20-year sex-appropriate WHO growth chart.

Pediatric Nutrition Handbook: An Algorithmic Approach, First Edition. Edited by David L. Suskind and Polly Lenssen.
© 2011 Blackwell Publishing Ltd. Published 2011 by Blackwell Publishing Ltd.

3. **Height-for-age:** A measure for chronic malnutrition.
4. **Reference:** Waterlow classification (1973): height-for-age.

Height deficit (%): (Actual height [cm] ÷ expected height at the 50th percentile for age) × 100	
Normal height	95–100%
Mildly stunted	90–95%
Moderately stunted	85–90%
Severely stunted	<85%

1.1.3 Weight-for-Length (Up to 36 Months)

Measure for acute malnutrition as well as obesity.

1. **Plot on a 0- to 36-month sex-appropriate WHO growth chart.**

High risk for underweight	<5th percentile
Moderate risk for underweight	<10th percentile
At risk for overweight	>85th percentile
Overweight	>95th percentile

1.1.4 Body Mass Index (BMI) in kg/m^2 (2–20 Years)

Measure for undernutrition and obesity.

1. **Calculate (k/m^2):** (weight in kg) ÷ (height in meters) ÷ (height in meters).
2. **Plot on a 2- to 20-year sex-appropriate WHO growth chart.**
3. **Interpretation:** Barlow SE; Expert Committee, 2007.

Underweight	<5th percentile
Healthy weight	5–84th percentile
Overweight	85–94th percentile
Obese	>95th percentile

1.1.5 Ideal Body Weight

1. **Methods:**
   a. Weight at which weight-for-length is 50th percentile for age (0–36 months) or BMI is 50th-percentile BMI for age (2–20 years).
   b. Weight at the 50th percentile at the age that matches the height-for-age.
2. **% Ideal body weight (IBW) = Actual weight/IBW.**

3. **Interpretation:** McLaren and Read, 1972.

Normal nutrition	90–109%
Mild malnutrition	85–89%
Moderate malnutrition	75–84%
Severe malnutrition	<75%

1.1.6 Growth Velocity or Incremental Growth

1. **Detect abnormal rates of growth or weight gain** before child is at extremes on growth chart; monitor efficacy of nutrition therapy.
2. **Infants 0–24 months:**
   a. Calculate weight gain in g/day and compare to standards: See Appendix A.
   b. Calculate linear growth in mm/day (cm/day × 100) and compare to standards. See Appendix B.
3. **Children 2–10 years:** Calculate weight gain in g/day and compare to standards listed here.

Expected Gain in Weight: >2 Years Old (Fomon et al., 1982)		
Age (years)	**Weight (g/day)**	**Weight (g/day)**
	Boys	**Girls**
2–3	5.7	6.0
3–4	5.5	5.1
4–5	5.4	4.7
5–6	5.5	5.1
6–7	5.9	6.4
7–8	6.7	8.2
8–9	7.8	9.9
9–10	9.1	11.2

1.1.7 Specialty Growth Charts

1. **Premature:** Plot for gestational age until 50 weeks; then correct for prematurity on standard WHO growth charts until 24 months.
2. **Charts for** achondroplasia, cerebral palsy, Down syndrome, Noonan syndrome, Prader-Willi syndrome, Turner syndrome, and Williams syndrome are available. Use in conjunction with standard WHO growth charts.

1.1.8 Occipital Frontal Circumference (0–36 months)

1. **Plot on sex-appropriate WHO growth charts.**
2. **Interpretation:**
   a. Rapid increase in rate of growth may indicate hydrocephalus.
   b. Decrease in rate of growth may indicate developmental delay; associated with malnutrition.
3. **Note if patient has a shunt.**

1.1.9   Arm Muscle and Fat Stores (>12 months)

1. **Use to detect serial changes in body composition;** only valid when repeat measurements are made by the same observer and interpreted over time.
2. **Measure mid-upper-arm circumference** (AC) and triceps skin fold thickness (TSF) and calculate arm area (AA), arm muscle area (AMA), and arm fat area (AFA).
   a. Calculations
      - AA (mm^2): (AC [mm])^2 ÷ 4π
      - AMA (mm^2): (AC [mm] − πTSF)^2 ÷ 4π
      - AFA (mm^2): AA − AMA.
3. **Compare to standards** (limitation: data from whites only). See Frisancho (1981).

1.1.10   Clinical Evaluation

1. **Nutritional status is affected** not only by the nutritional intake but also by developmental status, disease states, medications, and surgical/medical procedures.
2. **Symptoms that may affect adequacy of intake:** Vomiting, diarrhea, constipation, dysphagia, abnormal sucking or chewing, abdominal pain/gas, respiratory distress, heart failure, renal failure, and almost any chronic disease.
3. **Physical examination results:**
   a. Clinical signs in the malnourished child:
      - Marasmus: A form of severe malnutrition that occurs with total energy deficiency (i.e., "skin and bones").
      - Kwashiorkor: A form of malnutrition that occurs when there is not enough protein in the diet.
      Refer to Chapter 2, Section 2.10, for signs and symptoms of vitamin/mineral deficiency or excess.
   b. **Hydration status:**
      - Degrees and signs of dehydration in children (see table) (reference: Satter, 2000):

Degree of Dehydration	Symptoms
Mild dehydration (<3%)	• Slightly dry mouth • Increased thirst • Decreased urination
Moderate dehydration (3–6%)	• Sunken eyes • Sunken fontanelle • Skin not as smooth or elastic • Dry mouth • Few tears when child cries

Degree of Dehydration	Symptoms
Severe dehydration (>6%)	• Signs of moderate dehydration plus: • Rapid, light pulse • Unusually blue skin • Rapid breathing • Cold hands and feet • Listlessness, drowsiness • Loss of consciousness

Source: Copyright © 2011 by Ellyn Satter. Reproduced with permission from *Child of Mine: Feeding with Love and Good Sense*, Bull Publishing, Boulder, CO, 2000.

1.1.11   Laboratory Assessment

Many tests are affected by disease and fluid status, and they may not be useful for guiding nutrition therapy. Ask, "Will the results change the nutrition intervention strategy?" before requesting a test be ordered.

1. **Protein indices:**
   a. Albumin: Affected by fluid status, infection, or inflammation; long half-life (~23 days).
   b. Prealbumin, transferrin, retinal-binding protein: Depressed during stress, infection, and acute illness; shorter half-lives.
   c. C-reactive protein (CRP): Elevated during stress, infection, and inflammation; may be used with other protein indices to help determine whether low protein level is due to stress or nutritional status.
2. **Iron status:**
   a. Hemoglobin and/or hematocrit: Low only in later stages of iron deficiency anemia. May be low due to other disease states (renal failure, B_{12}, or folate deficiency, hematologic or cancer diagnoses) even with normal iron status.
   b. Ferritin: Indicative of iron status but elevated during infection or chronic inflammation.
   c. Total iron-binding capacity (TIBC); percentage saturation, serum iron: Use with ferritin to assess iron status.
3. **Immunologic function:**
   a. Total lymphocyte count: Depressed in malnutrition but also altered due to immunosuppressant drug therapy, chemotherapy or radiation, and/or trauma.
4. **Vitamin/mineral/trace element status:**
   a. Zinc: May be low secondary to inadequate intake, increased losses, or malabsorption.
   b. Vitamin A: May be low secondary to inadequate intake or fat malabsorption.
   c. Vitamin D: May be low secondary to inadequate intake, inadequate supplementation of high-risk patients, and/or fat malabsorption.

5. **Examples of disease or condition-specific labs in pediatric assessment:**
   a. Antiseizure medications: Serum calcium, phosphorus, alkaline phosphatase, and vitamin D.
   b. Poor growth in infants and young children: Serum bicarbonate.
   c. Phenylketonuria (PKU): Serum phenylalanine.
   d. Renal failure: Serum electrolytes, calcium, phosphorus, intact parathyroid hormone.
   e. Low energy needs: Selenium (to ensure adequate provision).
6. **Very low-fat diet (intestinal lymphangiectasia/chylothorax) or significantly elevated triglycerides preventing adequate parenteral fat provision:**
   a. Check essential fatty acid profile after 2 weeks and update every 1–3 months as indicated. Interpretation provided by Mayo Clinic with lab results.
7. **See total parenteral nutrition (TPN) guidelines for recommendations regarding lab monitoring for TPN patients.**

1.1.12 Dietary Evaluation

1. **Feeding problem history:** Chronological from birth or onset of current problem.
2. **Current intake:**
   a. Typical daily intake, food frequency, and/or food records.
   b. Breast-feeding infants: Frequency and duration of feedings, how much mother obtains if/when pumps, fullness of breasts pre- and postfeedings; for hospitalized infants, use pre- and postfeeding weights.
3. **Special diets:**
   a. Religious or cultural diet restrictions.
   b. Physician- or dietitian-prescribed therapeutic diets.
   c. Self-chosen lifestyle (e.g., vegetarian, milk free, etc.).
4. **Food allergies.**
5. **Nutrient supplements.**
6. **Complementary medicine** (self-prescribed or by alternative provider):
   a. Diet
   b. Herbal remedies
   c. Supplements
   d. Over-the-counter (OTC) products.

1.1.13 Physical Activity

1. **Usual activity or exercise.**
2. **"Inactivity"** (time spent with TV, video games, computer, reading, studying).
3. **Changes in activity** due to disease/condition.

1.1.14   Estimation of Nutrient Needs

1. **Energy** (reassess frequently to avoid over- or underfeeding):
   a. Estimated energy requirement (EER) for age, sex, weight, and physical activity coefficient. EER (kcal/day) = total energy expenditure + energy deposition.
   b. Basal metabolic rate × factor:
      - World Health Organization (WHO).

Age range (years)	kcal/day
Males	
0–3	(60.9 × weight [kg]) − 54
3–10	(22.7 × weight [kg]) + 495
10–18	(17.5 × weight [kg]) + 651
Females	
0–3	(61.0 × weight [kg]) − 51
3–10	(22.5 × weight [kg]) + 499
10–18	(12.2 × weight [kg]) + 746

   c. Basal energy expenditure (BEE) × factor (>18 years):
      - Harris-Benedict equation:

Females	BEE = 65.5 + (9.6 × weight [kg]) + (1.8 × height [cm]) − (4.7 × age [years])
Males	BEE = 66.5 + (13.7 × weight [kg]) + (5 × height [cm]) − (6.8 × age)

2. **Protein** (Recommended Daily Allowance [RDA] + increase or decrease for condition):

Life Stage Group	Protein (g/kg body weight)
0–6 months	1.52
7–12 months	1.2
1–3 years	1.05
4–13 years	0.95
14–18 years	0.85

3. **Fluid** (start with maintenance fluid requirements and increase or decrease based on clinical condition):

<10 kg	100 mL/kg
10–20 kg	1000 mL + 50 mL/kg for every kg above 10 kg
20–40 kg	1500 mL + 20 mL/kg for every kg above 20 kg
>40 kg	1500 mL per body surface area (m^2) (m^2 = square root [height in cm × weight in kg] ÷ 60)

4. **Vitamins and minerals:**
   a. DRI (Dietary Reference Intake): Adequate intake or RDA + increase or decrease for condition.
   b. Upper limit (UL) (tolerable upper intake levels) for safe UL.

1.2 Focused Assessment: Infants
Cheryl Davis and the Clinical Nutrition Department

1.2.1 Anthropometrics and Growth Assessment

1. **Compare rate of weight gain and linear growth** to expected rates for age. See the growth assessment tables in the General Pediatric Nutrition Assessment section.
   a. Measure weight daily and length weekly.
2. **Former premature:** Correct on growth chart for prematurity until 24 months.

1.2.2 Dietary Assessment

1. **24-recall, 3-day food record** or direct observation.
2. **Eating behavior history:**
   a. Initial form of nourishment.
   b. Who feeds infant?
   c. Does infant feed differently for different feeders?
   d. Any formula changes? What formulas specifically used, how long and why changed?
   e. How long does a feeding take? How much per feeding?
   f. Formula preparation?
   g. Symptoms: Any diarrhea, vomiting, or constipation?
   h. Any arching back during or after feeding?
   i. Does milk or formula drip out of mouth while infant is feeding?
   j. Is infant or mother on Women, Infants and Children (Nutritional Program) (WIC)? Does family run out of formula before next WIC appointment?
   k. Have solid foods been introduced? If so, at what age?
3. **Vitamin D supplementation:** Per American Academy of Pediatrics (AAP) recommendations, all infants should have a supplement of 400 IU/day beginning during the first 2 months of life through childhood and adolescence unless ingesting at least 500 mL/day of vitamin D–fortified formula or milk.
4. **Fluoride supplementation:** Per AAP recommendations, infants ≥6 months should supplement with 0.25 mg/day in areas with <0.3 ppm fluoride concentration in community drinking supplies.

5. **Expected feeding capabilities for age** (see table).
6. **Reference:** Satter, 2000 (see table).

Age	Skills	Suggested Foods
Birth–6 months	• Cuddles, roots for nipple • Sucks and swallows	• Breast milk, formula
5–7 months	• Sits supported with head control • Follows food with eyes • Opens mouth for spoon • Closes lips over spoon • Moves semisolids to the back of tongue • Swallows semisolids	• Breast milk, formula • Iron-fortified cereals
6–8 months	• Sits alone • Keeps food in mouth • Pushes food to jaws with tongue • Munches/mashes food with up-and-down movement • Palmar grasp • Scrapes food from hand to mouth • Drinks from cup (but loses a lot)	• Breast milk, formula • Mashed/pureed fruits and vegetables • Pureed meats
7–10 months	• Sits alone easily • Chews with rotary motion • Bites off food • Moves food side to side in mouth • Begins curving lips around cup • Pincer grasp	• Breast milk, formula • Chopped cooked vegetables and fruits • Mashed cooked beans • Strips of bread, toast, tortillas • Crackers and dried cereals
7–10 months	• Sits alone easily • Chews with rotary motion • Bites off food • Moves food side to side in mouth • Begins curving lips around cup • Pincer grasp	• Breast milk, formula • Chopped cooked vegetables and fruits • Mashed cooked beans • Strips of bread, toast, tortillas • Crackers and dried cereals
9–12 months	• Pincer grasp improves • Curves lips around cup • Getting better at controlling food in mouth • Getting better at chewing	• Breast milk, formula • Cut-up soft cooked foods • Cut-up soft raw fruits • Tender chopped/mashed meats • Dry cereal, toast, crackers • Eggs and cheese
>12 months	• Becomes more skillful with hands • Finger-feeds • Improves chewing • Improves cup drinking • Is interested in food	• Whole milk • Soft foods from family table

Source: Copyright © 2011 by Ellyn Satter. Reproduced with permission from *Child of Mine: Feeding with Love and Good Sense*, Bull Publishing, Boulder, CO, 2000.

Practical recommendations for initiating complementary foods (American Academy of Pediatrics 2009; used with permission of the American Academy of Pediatrics, *Pediatric Nutrition Handbook*, 6th edition, (c) 2009 American Academy of Pediatrics):

- Introduce one single-ingredient food at a time to identify possible allergic reactions.
- Choose foods that provide key nutrients, such as iron and zinc.
- Introduce a variety of foods by the end of the first year.
- Withhold cow's milk (and other milk substitutes not formulated for infants) during the first year of life.
- Ensure adequate calcium intake when transitioning to complementary foods.
- Do not introduce juice during the first 6 months of life.
- Ensure safe ingestion and adequate nutrition when choosing and preparing homemade foods.
- Choking hazards: Whole grapes, hot dog rounds, raisins, raw carrots, nuts, and round candies.

1.2.3   Estimation of Nutrient Needs

1. **Energy and protein:** See the equations for estimating energy and protein needs in the General Pediatric Nutrition Assessment section.
2. **Fluids:** See the General Pediatric Nutrition Assessment section.

1.2.4   Nutrition Intervention

1. **Underweight infants:** Nutrition intervention is critical because primary and secondary malnutrition can result in irreversible sequelae:
   a. Assess feeding volumes and frequency. Calculate average daily intake and compare to estimated needs.
   b. Boost overall calorie intake:
      - Increase caloric density of breast milk or formula (concentrate formula).
      - Possible change in formula based on diagnosis or tolerance.
      - Possible change in route of nourishment, including supplemental tube feedings.
      - Possible change in viscosity of formula (if ascending or descending aspiration).
   c. One-on-one intervention with caregivers:
      - Lactation expert.
      - Parenting classes.
      - Public health nurse referral.
      - Education on feeding techniques.
      - Financial referrals (WIC, food stamps, Supplemental Security Income [SSI]).
      - Review of OTC products and safety.

2. **Overweight infants** (gaining >35 g/day or weight for length >95th percentile): A growth-suppressed infant may need calories adjusted based on weight gain, growth, and clinical response:
   a. Decrease volume or density of formula.
   b. Analyze for micronutrients to ensure adequate provision with reduced formula provision.

1.3 Focused Assessment: Toddlers

Cheryl Davis and the Clinical Nutrition Department

1.3.1 Anthropometrics and Growth Assessment

1. **Monitoring:**
   a. Inpatient:
      - Weight 2 to 3× per week.
      - Height every 2–4 weeks.
   b. Outpatient:
      - Weight weekly if severely malnourished or medically fragile; every other week if moderately malnourished.
      - Height every 2–4 weeks.
2. **Expected rate of weight gain:** Compare actual rate of gain to standard for age (see the growth assessment tables in the General Pediatric Nutrition Assessment section).
3. **Expected rate length or stature gain:** Compare actual rate of linear growth/stature to standard for age (see the growth assessment tables in the General Pediatric Nutrition Assessment section).

1.3.2 Dietary and Eating Behavior Assessment

1. **24-hour diet recall and food frequency.**
2. **Eating behavior history:**

Age	Eating Behavior History
0–4 months	• Breast- or formula-fed? • If formula, preparation? • Feed frequency?
4–6 months	• When and what were first solids? • Reaction to solids by spoon? • Frequency of solids? • Any change in breast-feeding or bottle intake? • When introduced to juice or water? • Approximately how much juice and water? • Any problems?

Age	Eating Behavior History
6–10 months	• When did child transition to finger foods? • What finger foods did child eat? • Frequency of finger foods? • Approximate volume of formula, juice and/or water? • Any change in breast-feeding or bottle intake?
10–12 months	• Was child spoon-feeding or taking finger foods? • Where did child eat solids? • How were solids and fluids coordinated? • Feeding frequency? • Any structure? • Juice, water volume per day? • Any feeds at night?
12+ months	• Is child breast-feeding or on formula? • Has child been introduced to cow's milk? • Frequency of solids and beverages? • Any structure to day? • Any change in milk, juice, or water volume from 12 mo to present age? • Has child ever taken concentrated formula or supplement? • Has child ever been prescribed vitamins?

3. **Three-day food record:**
   a. Compare intake of kcal, protein, vitamins, and minerals to needs.
   b. Assess timing of meals and snacks.
   c. Assess balance of fluids and solids.
   d. Assess balance of milk/milk alternatives to juice, water, gelatin, broth, and other lower calorie fluids.
4. **Common contributors to inadequate nutrient intake:**
   a. Inadequate and inconsistent feeding frequency (<5 to 6×/day).
   b. Grazing: Solids and fluids offered >6×/day and/or solids and fluids not coordinated such that 2–3 hours do not pass between meals and snacks to gain an optimal appetite.
   c. **Excessive juice and/or water intake** (AAP recommends an upper limit of 4–6 oz).
   d. **Imbalanced solid/fluid intake:**
      • <16–24 oz milk or equivalent daily and/or solids representing >60–70% of total energy intake.
      • >24 oz milk and other fluids daily and/or solids representing <40–50% of total energy intake.
   e. **Frequent intake of low-fat, low-nutrient-dense foods** (i.e., >3–4 servings of fresh fruit, vegetables, gelatin, broth soup, rice cakes, saltine crackers) and low intake of high-fat foods from starch, dairy, and protein groups.
   f. **Inadequate intake:**
      • "Bites" and "sips" of food and fluid offered.
      • Behavioral issues strong enough that the child's need to control overrides hunger cues.

- Psychosocial issues such as anxiety or loneliness that override hunger cues.

g. **Breast-feeding not coordinated** with solid and other fluid intake such that overall feeding frequency >6×/day results in decreased appetite.

h. **Preoccupation with breast-feeding beyond infancy:** Child shows little interest in solids or fluids other than breast milk, creating an imbalance of calories from solids and fluids. This is most concerning after 8–10 months when transition to finger foods usually takes place and energy and nutrient needs from solids increase.

i. **Continued use of baby food textures as primary diet** past 10–12 months.

j. **Continued use of bottle.**

k. **Typical portion sizes for toddlers 1–3 years.** See table (Satter, 1987).

Food	Typical Portion Size for Toddler
Meat, poultry, fish	1–2 Tbsp
Eggs	¼ egg
Cooked dried beans	1–2 Tbsp
Pasta, rice, potatoes	1–2 Tbsp
Bread	¼ slice
Vegetables	1–2 Tbsp
Fruit	1–2 Tbsp or ¼ piece
Milk	¼–⅓ cup

Note: Children may eat more or less, but this is how much you can serve them to start with.
Source: Copyright © 2011 by Ellyn Satter. Reproduced with permission from *How to Get Your Kid to Eat – But Not Too Much*. Bull Publishing, Boulder, CO, 1987.

1.3.3   Estimation of Nutrient Needs

1. **Proportional growth/weight gain:**
   a. Energy and protein: See the equations for estimating energy and protein needs in the General Pediatric Nutrition Assessment section.
2. **Catch-up weight gain/repletion:**
   a. Energy:
      - Basal metabolic rate (BMR) (based on IBW) × 1.8 to 2.
   b. Protein (dependent on disease state and level of depletion):
      - 1.2–1.5 g/kg if:
        - No disease process.
        - Oral protein intake is lower than RDA.
        - Mild protein store depletion.
      - 1.2–2.0 g/kg if:
        - High protein turnover (disease, trauma or medication).
        - Oral protein intake meets RDA and stores are still depleted.
3. **Fluid** (see the General Pediatric Nutrition Assessment section).

4. Risk of nutrient deficiency in this age group per the American Academy of Pediatrics (2009):
   a. Iron.
   b. Calcium and vitamin D.
   c. Vitamin A.
   d. Zinc.

1.3.4   Nutrition Intervention

1. **Oral intake:**
   a. Structured meals and snacks every 2–3 hours 6×/day.
   b. If continued breast-feeding, coordinate to follow directly after meals/snacks.
   c. Fluid intake:
      - Meets 40–50% of estimated energy needs.
      - 16–24 oz milk or equivalent.
      - Juice maximum 4–6 oz/day.
   d. Solids meet 40–50% estimated energy needs.
   e. Avoid potential choking hazards:

Potential Choking Hazards for Toddlers		
Hot dogs	Chunks of meat	Nuts
Peanut butter	Raw apples	Raw carrots
Corn	Grapes	Popcorn
Hand candy	Jellybeans	Gumdrops

1.3.5   Mealtime Duties

Ellyn Satter describes the Division of Responsibility in feeding between parents and children (see Satter 1987, 2000).

1. It is the role of the parent to provide age-appropriate foods with scheduled meals and snacks in a consistent place (e.g., at the table versus in front of the TV). Family meals are encouraged.
2. It is the role of the child to determine whether or not to eat the provided food.

1.3.6   Weight Gain

If concerned about poor weight gain, may consider supplementation with high-calorie foods and drinks:

- If food fails, try a commercial oral supplement such as PediaSure, Nutren Junior, Boost Kid Essentials, or Bright Beginnings.
- Whole milk with Instant Breakfast powder drink mix.
- Regular or vanilla-flavored soy milk plus Polycose or Duocal.
- Whole milk with Ovaltine drink mix.
- Whole-milk yogurt.
- Milkshakes.

1.3.7   Additional Feedings

Tube feedings may be indicated if oral intake is inadequate to meet needs.

1.4   Focused Assessment: School-Age Children
Cheryl Davis and the Clinical Nutrition Department

1.4.1   Anthropometrics and Growth

1. **Monitoring:**
   a. Inpatient:
      - Weight weekly: If concerned about malnutrition or fluid-sensitive issues, weight can be checked daily or twice a day.
      - Height monthly.
   b. Outpatient (if concerns for poor growth):
      - Weight: 1× month.
      - Height: 1–4×/year.
2. **Expected rate of weight gain:** Compare actual rate of gain to standard for age (see the growth assessment tables in the General Pediatric Nutrition Assessment section).

1.4.2   Diet History and Eating Behavior Characteristics

1. **24-hour recall and food frequency.**
2. **Patient and family interview:**
   a. Who does child eat with?
   b. How many meals are eaten at school?
   c. What are sources of nutrition information (school, parent, media)?
   d. Are parents overweight? Dieting?
3. **Characteristics that influence eating behavior:**
   a. Growing independence may lead to:
      - Resistance to certain foods and food groups.
      - Transfer of control of food selection from parent to child.
      - Preparation and/or purchase of snacks by child, not parent.

   b. Involvement in other activities may result in failure to respond to internal eating cues.
4. **Reference:** Satter, 2000 (see table).

	Typical Portion Sizes for Age		
Food	**Ages 3–5 years**	**Ages 6–8 years**	**Ages 8+ years**
Meat, poultry, fish	1 oz	1–2 oz	2 oz
Eggs	½ egg	¾ egg	1 egg
Cooked dried beans	3–5 Tbsp	5–8 Tbsp	½ cup
Pasta, rice, potatoes	3–5 Tbsp	5–8 Tbsp	½ cup
Bread	½ slice	1 slice	1 slice
Vegetables	3–5 Tbsp	5–8 Tbsp	½ cup
Fruit	3–5 Tbsp or ⅓ piece	5–8 Tbsp or ½ piece	½ cup or 1 piece
Milk	⅓–½ cup	½–⅔ cup	1 cup

Note: Children may eat more or less, but this is how much you can serve them to start with.
Source: Copyright © 2011 by Ellyn Satter. Reproduced with permission from *Child of Mine: Feeding with Love and Good Sense*, Bull Publishing, Boulder, CO, 2000.

1.4.3   Estimation of Nutrient Needs

1. **Normal weight gain:**
   a. Energy and protein: See the equations for estimating energy and protein needs in the General Pediatric Nutrition Assessment section.
2. **Catch-up growth:**
   a. Energy:
      • BMR × 1.8 to 2.
      • 90–100 kcal/kg.
      • 17–20 kcal/cm.
   b. Protein: 1.5–1.8 g/kg.
3. **Slow weight velocity for weight management:** BMR (based on IBW) × 1.3–1.5.
4. **Fluid:** See the General Pediatric Nutrition Assessment section.
5. **Risk of nutrient deficiency in this age group per the American Academy of Pediatrics (2009):** Calcium, vitamin D, vitamin A, iron, zinc, magnesium, and vitamin B_6.
6. **General nutrition guidelines for children (American Academy of Pediatrics 2009) (used with permission of the American Academy of Pediatrics, *Pediatric Nutrition Handbook*, 6th edition, (c) 2009 American Academy of Pediatrics):**
   a. Make available and offer a colorful variety of fruits and vegetables for children to consume every day.
   b. Limit intake of foods and beverages with added sugar or salt.
   c. Keep total fat between 25% and 35% of total calories for children 4–18 years of age.
   d. Offer fruits, vegetables, fat-free or low-fat dairy, and whole-grain snacks.
   e. Offer child-appropriate portions.

f. Engage in at least 60 minutes of moderate to vigorous physical activity on most, if not all, days of the week.

g. Provide food that is safe (avoid unpasteurized milk/juices and raw or undercooked meat, poultry, eggs, fish, and shellfish).

1.4.4 Intervention

1. **Underweight:**
   a. High-calorie-diet education.
   b. High-calorie oral supplements (see the Toddlers section).
   c. Supplemental tube feeding if indicated.
2. **Overweight/obese:**
   a. Family-based behavior change.
   • Portion control, family meals, healthy snacks, beverage choices, physical activity.
3. **Picky eating:**
   a. Division of responsibility (see the Toddlers section).

1.5 Focused Assessment: Adolescents
Alicia Dixon Docter

1.5.1 Introduction

The onset of puberty presents increased nutrition risk due to dramatic changes in physical, cognitive, and emotional development.

1.5.2 Nutrient Needs

1. **There is an increased demand for most nutrients** due to pronounced linear growth and increases in muscle mass, vascular system, adipose layers, and bone density. At the same time, lifestyle changes – increased reliance on peers, greater independence in food choice, availability and increased activity – add complexity to helping adolescents meet their needs. Feeding behaviors have been developing since teens were babies. In an ideal situation, teens will be able gradually to individuate and begin to meet their nutrition needs. Special situations in which additional guidance is needed:
   a. Vigorous sports and physical training; female athlete triad.
   b. Excessive dieting.
   c. Eating disorders.
   d. Obesity.
   e. Pregnancy.
   f. Drug and alcohol use.
   g. Lifestyle diets (e.g., vegetarian).
   h. Chronic illness.

2. **Primary risks of undernutrition:**
   a. Delayed puberty.
   b. Amenorrhea.
   c. Decreased bone mineralization.
   d. Bradycardia/tachycardia.
   e. Growth stunting.
   f. Iron deficiency.
   g. Dehydration.
3. **Energy needs:**
   a. Energy needs correlate more to pubertal growth spurt than chronological age. Additionally, energy needs vary between individuals due to differences in growth velocity, age of puberty, proportion of lean body mass to adipose tissue, and physical activity. Estimates of needs can be reassessed when compared to nutrient intake, weight gain and growth over a 1- to 3-month period.
   b. Males: Energy needs accelerate with the onset of puberty (i.e., heightened linear growth and weight gain) due to a twofold increase in muscle mass. Peak velocity of linear growth occurs later in puberty among males than females (14.4 years on average).
   c. Females: Peak velocity of linear growth takes place ~6–12 months prior to menarche (average age of menarche is 12.5 years). Weight gain slows around the time of menarche but continues into late adolescence. By 18 years of age, >90% of adult skeletal mass has been accrued. Adequate energy intake and growth are essential to support normal menstruation, which will in turn support development of peak bone mass.
   d. Calculating energy needs:
      • Energy goal for weight gain: BMR (based on IBW for height) × 1.5–1.7 kcal.
      • Energy goal for weight loss: BMR (based on IBW for height) × 1.3–1.5 kcal.
4. **Protein needs:**
   a. DRI for age allows for needs during the most accelerated adolescent growth period (i.e., no need to adjust for growth and age of maturation).
   b. Protein should constitute ~20% of total energy, which is generally achieved with eating normal meals and snacks at the estimated goal energy level.
   c. Protein needs for competitive athletes to support tissue repair and red blood cell synthesis during extensive muscle building and strength training may be as high as 150–200% × DRI or 1.2–1.5 g/kg.
5. **Vitamins and minerals:**
   RDI for age allows for nutrient needs during the most accelerated adolescent growth period (i.e., no need to adjust for growth and age of maturation). Typical adolescent eating patterns or chronic disease can set teens up for the following nutrient concerns:

a. Iron deficiency: Prevalent and significant for both genders, all races, and all socioeconomic levels (National Health and Nutrition Examination II Survey). Iron is required for adequate developmental growth and immune function. For a diagnosed deficiency, conduct a thorough history and consider the following:
  - Assessment of bioavailability of iron sources and vitamin C intake.
  - Supplement 325 mg $FeSO_4$ by mouth 3x/day for 2–3 months. Repeat iron indices to assess repletion.
  - Sports anemia in adolescent athletes: A transient decrease in hemoglobin due to increased erythrocyte destruction as a result of an acute response to exercise and training.

b. Folate deficiency: Increased needs coupled with poor to variable fruit and vegetable intake may lead to deficiency. Explore intake and acceptable food choices (e.g., fresh orange or tangerine juice and fortified cereals).

c. Calcium and vitamin D: Increased risk of osteopenia and osteoporosis with chronic steroid treatment and energy deficit related to secondary amenorrhea.

6. **Fluid:**
a. General: See the General Pediatric Nutrition Assessment section.
b. Exercise: Physically untrained teens are at risk for dehydration and heatstroke and require more fluids to maintain hydration and temperature regulation than physically trained teens. Untrained individuals should have unlimited access to fluids during exercise to improve hydration and temperature regulation. Fluid loss representing a 2% decrease in body weight may impede strength and stamina:
  - Exercise <60 minutes: Water is recommended for fluid replacement.
  - Exercise >60 minutes: Sports drinks containing 6–8% carbohydrate (50–80 kcal/8 oz) are recommended to supply energy and electrolyte replacement for optimal fluid absorption (>10% carbohydrate kcal slows fluid absorption; <5% carbohydrate kcal supplies inadequate energy).

1.5.3   Assessment

1. **Physical parameters:**
a. Weight, height, and BMI:
  - Plot current data on a sex-appropriate CDC chart (2–20 years).
  - Compare with weight and height history to determine change in weight and growth velocity past 3–12 months.
  - Adjusted body weight (used in some chemotherapy dosing) = IBW + 0.25 (actual weight − IBW).
b. IBW: Estimate based on available growth history; generally between the 25th and 75th percentile for BMI-for-age.

    c. Interpretation and goals:
- General weight goal is 90–110% IBW.
- Rapid or chronic weight loss to ≤85–90% IBW increases risk of delayed puberty or amenorrhea; sustained weight >90% IBW for several months is the goal for menses to resume.

    d. Monitoring weight and height:
- Inpatient: One to three times per week depending on acuity of condition.
- Outpatient: Weekly to biweekly until stable lifestyle, oral intake, and weight goals are demonstrated; then monthly to every 2–6 months as needed to demonstrate progress toward and achievement of goals.
- Height: Check monthly to demonstrate compliance with weight goals; then every 2–6 months as needed with weight checks.

    e. Arm muscle and fat stores measured by the registered dietitian:
- Estimate body type (endomorph, ectomorph, or mesomorph).
- General goal is 25–75th percentile for age and sex.
- Assess every 6–8 weeks as needed to demonstrate body composition changes.
- Can be a very helpful *educational* tool (e.g., high amount of muscle mass may explain high BMI).

2. **Patient and family interview:**

    a. Identify nutrition risks and intervention opportunities related to the patients' goals, eating behaviors, and attitudes toward health.

    b. Evaluation of weight history, body image, and self-esteem:
- What are the concerns of patients and their families? Do they differ?
- Has weight changed in the past 6–12 months? Highest? Lowest? When?
- What weight do patients wish to be?
- What weight do patients view as "healthy"?
- How have patients tried to achieve their desired or healthy weight?
- Have patients changed the way they eat in the past 6–12 months?
- Have patients tried vomiting, diet pills, or laxatives to change weight? What were the results?
- What are the patients' activity levels? Has this changed in the last 6–12 months?

    c. Dietary evaluation:
- Obtain a 24-hour recall and best description of meal frequency.
- Where and with whom is each meal eaten?
- Who prepares the food most often?
- Are meals skipped? How many times per week?
- Are patients regularly omitting one or more major food groups?
- Do patients ever eat large amounts of food that they wish they had not? Alone or with a friend?
- Have patients ever felt it was hard to stop eating?
- Are meals consumed on the run or while doing other activities (e.g., TV, at work, on the bus)?
- Do patients take vitamins or other nutritional supplements?
- Is there drug, alcohol, tobacco, or caffeine use?

d. Perceived family health history:
- Are patients aware of any health problems in their families?
- Does anyone in the family need to follow a special diet or has anyone attempted a weight loss diet in the past?
- Where have patients gained health and nutrition knowledge?

3. **Laboratory:**
   a. Serum vitamin A (vitamin A required for reproductive development) when there is delayed puberty and marginal vitamin A intake by history.
   b. Serum lipid levels when BMI >85th percentile, diet history is significant for high fat, and patient symptomatic for health problems related to obesity.
   c. Serum calcium, vitamin D, and alkaline phosphatase when calcium intake by history is low, patient is amenorrheic, or has taken steroid medications for >1 month.

1.5.4 Approaches to Communication with Adolescents in Nutrition Intervention

1. **Keep the adolescent's psychosocial and cognitive development in mind.** There are three periods: early (11–14 years), middle (15–17 years), and late (18–21 years).
2. **Generally, younger teens are more concrete in their thinking.** As they get older, they are able to manage more abstract concepts as well as become more independent of parents in terms of decision making. At all stages, peers have a very strong effect on their decision making, yet studies show that parents continue to be an influence even as their children become more independent.
3. **Develop rapport** using Motivational Interviewing (MI) tools such as open-ended questions, reflective listening, and affirmations. MI has been found to be effective in communicating with adolescents.
4. **Ask to identify their perceptions** of why they are meeting with you and their perceived needs for treatment. Use information to confirm patient knowledge/awareness and as a starting point for nutrition/physiologic education.
5. **Ask teens what "healthy," "healthy nutrition," or "healthy activity" means to them;** it is also a good starting point for nutrition and physiologic education.
6. **Adolescents are typically well educated with respect to "healthy" food choices or calories** but often have a distorted sense of regular eating frequency, meal and snack patterns, and appetite/satiety awareness.
7. **Avoid judgment.** Portray ultimate respect for the teens' development and struggle for self-confidence, individuality, and social acceptance. The MI concept of "rolling with resistance" can be helpful in sessions where teens are struggling verbally.

8. **Expect experimentation with varied eating behaviors** to achieve social acceptance. Help teens identify the pros and cons of less healthy choices and give specific reasons to prioritize health.
9. **Connect education** to life goals or to a physiologic event or development stage that the teen cares about, such as continued linear growth, puberty, appearance, immune function, muscle mass development, strong bones, academic achievement, or having fun with friends.
10. **Avoid making choices or giving ultimatums to teens.** Instead, recognize what they are doing well and provide education and recommendations for patients to consider when making their own food choices.
11. **In the context of specific education about nutrition and physiology, ask teens to identify one or two goals** they are willing to work on over a specified period of time to improve health. Give examples to choose from if needed.
12. **Provide written materials to both teens and families** if possible and appropriate.
13. **Respect teens' wishes for independence and privacy** from parents as desired. Ask teens if there are acceptable ways that parents can help them meet goals.

References

American Academy of Pediatrics Committee on Nutrition. *Pediatric Nutrition Handbook*. 6th ed. Elk Grove Village, IL: American Academy of Pediatrics; 2009.

Avencena IT, Cleghorn G. The nature and extent of malnutrition in children. In: Preedy VR, Grimble G, Watson R, eds. *Nutrition in the Infant: Problems and Practical Procedures*. Cambridge, UK: Cambridge University Press; 2008.

Barlow SE, Expert Committee. Expert committee recommendations regarding the prevention, assessment, and treatment of child and adolescent overweight and obesity: summary report. *Pediatrics*. 2007;120(4 Suppl):S164–S192.

Bessler S. Nutritional assessment. In: Samour PQ, King K, eds. *Handbook of Pediatric Nutrition*. 3rd ed. Sudbury, MA: Jones and Bartlett; 2005.

Centers for Disease Control and Prevention, National Center for Health Statistics. *CDC Growth Charts: United States*. http://www.cdc.gov/growthcharts/. May 2000.

Fomon SJ, Haschke F, Ziegler EE, Nelson SE. Body composition of reference children from birth to age 10 years. *Am J Clin Nutr*. 1982;35(5 Suppl):1169–1175.

Food and Nutrition Board of the Institute of Medicine of the National Academies. Dietary Reference Intake (DRI) reference tables. http://fnic.nal.usda.gov/nal_display/index.php?info_center=4&tax_level=3&tax_subject=256&topic_id=1342&level3_id=5140&level4_id=0&level5_id=0&placement_default=0.

Food and Nutrition Board of the Institute of Medicine of the National Academies. *Dietary Reference Intakes for Calcium, Phosphorus, Magnesium, Vitamin D and Fluoride*. Washington, DC: National Academies Press; 1999.

Food and Nutrition Board of the Institute of Medicine of the National Academies. *Dietary Reference Intakes for Energy, Carbohydrate, Fiber, Fat, Fatty Acids, Cholesterol, Protein and Amino Acids (Macronutrients)*. Washington, DC: National Academies Press; 2005.

Food and Nutrition Board of the Institute of Medicine of the National Academies. *Dietary Reference Intakes for Thiamin, Riboflavin, Niacin, Vitamin B6, Folate,*

Vitamin B12, Pantothenic Acid, Biotin and Choline. Washington, DC: National Academies Press; 1998.

Food and Nutrition Board of the Institute of Medicine of the National Academies. *Dietary Reference Intakes for Vitamin A, Vitamin K, Arsenic, Boron, Chromium, Copper, Iodine, Iron, Manganese, Molybdenum, Nickel, Silicon, Vanadium and Zinc*. Washington, DC: National Academies Press; 2001.

Food and Nutrition Board of the Institute of Medicine of the National Academies. *Dietary Reference Intakes for Vitamin C, Vitamin E, Selenium and Carotenoids*. Washington, DC: National Academies Press. 2000.

Frisancho AR. New norms of upper limb fat and muscle areas for assessment of nutritional status. *Am J Clin Nutr*. 1981;34(11):2540–2545.

Gómez F, Ramos GR, Frenk S, Cravioto-Muñoz J, Chávez R, Vázquez J. Mortality in second and third degree malnutrition. *J Trop Pediatr*. 1956;2(2):77–83.

Guo SM, Roche AF, Fomon SJ, et al. Reference data on gains in weight and length during the first two years of life. *J Pediatr*. 1991;119(3):355–362.

Harris JA, Benedict FG. *A Biometric Study of Basal Metabolism in Man*. Washington, DC: Carnegie Institute of Washington; 1919.

McLaren DS, Read WW. Classification of nutritional status in early childhood. *Lancet*. 1972;2(7769):146–148.

Nardella M, Campo L, Ogata B, eds. *Nutrition Interventions for Children with Special Health Care Needs*. 2nd ed. DOH Publication Number 961-158. Olympia, WA: Washington State Department of Health; 2002.

Rodríguez G, Moreno LA, Sarría A, Fleta J, Bueno M. Resting energy expenditure in children and adolescents: agreement between calorimetry and prediction equations. *Clin Nutr*. 2000;21(3):255–260.

Samour PQ, King K, eds. *Handbook of Pediatric Nutrition*. 3rd ed. Sudbury, MA: Jones and Bartlett; 2005.

Satter E. *Child of Mine: Feeding with Love and Good Sense*. 3rd ed. Boulder, CO: Bull Publishing; 2000.

Satter E. *How to Get Your Kid to Eat – But Not Too Much*. Boulder, CO: Bull Publishing; 1987.

Schofield W. Predicting basal metabolic rate, new standards and review of previous work. *Hum Nutr Clin Nutr*. 1985;39(1 Suppl):5–41.

Trumbo P, Schlicker S, Yates AA, Poos M; Food and Nutrition Board of the Institute of Medicine, The National Academies. Dietary reference intakes for energy, carbohydrate, fiber, fat, fatty acids, cholesterol, protein and amino acids. *J Am Diet Assoc*. 2002;102(11):1621–1630.

Waterlow JC. Note on the assessment and classification of protein-energy malnutrition in children. *Lancet*. 1973;2(7820):87–89.

Wong WW, Butte NF, Hergenroeder AC, Hill RB, Stuff JE, Smith EO. Are basal metabolic rate prediction equations appropriate for female children and adolescents? *J Apply Physiol*. 1996;81(6):2407–2414.

World Health Organization (WHO). *Energy and Protein Requirements*. Technical Report Series 724. Geneva, Switzerland: WHO; 1985.

Appendix A: Expected Gain in Weight: Birth to 24 Months (Guo et al., 1991)

Age (month)	N	Weight (g/day)	Percentile						
			5th	10th	25th	50th	75th	90th	95th
Boys									
Up to 3	580	31 ± 5.9	21	23	27	31	34	38	41
1–4	65	27 ± 5.1	–	21	23	27	30	34	–
2–5	65	21 ± 4.3	–	15	17	21	23	27	–
3–6	298	18 ± 2.9	13	14	16	18	19	21	23
4–7	233	16 ± 2.4	12	13	14	15	17	18	19
5–8	233	14 ± 2.4	11	11	13	14	15	17	18
6–9	233	13 ± 2.4	10	10	11	13	14	16	17
7–10	233	12 ± 2.4	9	9	10	12	13	15	16
8–11	233	11 ± 2.4	8	9	10	11	12	14	15
9–12	233	11 ± 2.3	8	8	9	10	12	14	14
10–13	233	10 ± 2.3	7	8	9	10	11	13	14
11–14	233	10 ± 2.3	7	7	8	9	11	12	13
12–15	233	9 ± 2.3	6	7	8	9	10	12	13
13–16	233	9 ± 9.3	6	6	7	9	10	12	13
14–17	233	8 ± 2.2	6	6	7	8	10	11	12
15–18	233	8 ± 2.2	5	6	7	8	9	11	12
16–19	233	8 ± 2.2	5	6	7	8	9	10	12
17–20	233	8 ± 2.2	5	5	6	7	9	10	12
18–21	233	7 ± 2.2	5	5	6	7	8	10	11
19–22	233	7 ± 2.1	4	5	6	7	8	10	11
20–23	233	7 ± 2.1	4	5	6	7	8	9	11
21–24	233	7 ± 2.1	4	5	6	7	8	9	11

Age (month)	N	Weight (g/day)	Percentile						
			5th	10th	25th	50th	75th	90th	95th
Girls									
Up to 3	562	26 ± 5.5	17	20	23	26	30	33	36
1–3	74	24 ± 5.1	–	19	21	24	27	30	–
2–5	74	20 ± 3.9	–	16	17	19	21	25	–
3–6	298	17 ± 4.6	12	13	15	17	18	20	21
4–7	224	15 ± 4.8	11	12	13	15	16	17	18
5–8	224	14 ± 4.7	10	11	12	13	15	16	17
6–9	224	13 ± 4.6	10	10	11	12	14	15	16
7–10	224	12 ± 4.5	9	9	10	12	13	14	15
8–11	224	11 ± 4.4	8	9	10	11	12	14	14
9–12	224	11 ± 4.3	8	8	9	10	12	13	14
10–13	224	10 ± 4.2	7	8	9	10	11	12	13

Age (month)	N	Weight (g/day)	Percentile						
			5th	10th	25th	50th	75th	90th	95th
11–14	224	10 ± 4.2	7	7	8	9	11	12	13
12–15	224	9 ± 4.1	7	7	8	9	10	12	12
13–16	224	9 ± 4.0	6	7	8	8	10	11	12
14–17	224	9 ± 3.9	6	6	7	8	9	11	12
15–18	224	8 ± 3.9	6	6	7	8	9	10	11
16–19	224	8 ± 3.8	6	6	7	8	9	10	11
17–20	224	8 ± 3.8	5	6	7	7	9	10	11
18–21	224	8 ± 3.7	5	5	6	7	8	10	11
19–22	224	7 ± 3.6	5	5	6	7	8	9	10
20–23	224	7 ± 3.6	5	5	6	7	8	9	10
21–24	224	7 ± 3.5	5	5	6	7	8	9	10

Appendix B: Expected Gain in Length: Birth to 24 Months (Guo et al., 1991)

Age (month)	N	Length (mm/day)	Percentile						
			5th	10th	25th	50th	75th	90th	95th
Boys									
Up to 3	580	1.07 ± 0.11	0.89	0.92	0.99	1.06	1.14	1.21	1.26
1–4	65	1.00 ± 0.08	–	0.90	0.94	1.01	1.06	1.09	–
2–5	65	0.84 ± 0.09	–	0.74	0.79	0.84	0.91	0.95	–
3–6	255	0.69 ± 0.08	0.56	0.60	0.64	0.68	0.73	0.79	0.82
4–7	190	0.62 ± 0.06	0.54	0.55	0.58	0.61	0.65	0.69	0.72
5–8	190	0.56 ± 0.05	0.49	0.50	0.53	0.56	0.59	0.63	0.65
6–9	190	0.52 ± 0.05	0.46	0.46	0.49	0.52	0.54	0.58	0.60
7–10	190	0.48 ± 0.05	0.42	0.43	0.45	0.48	0.51	0.54	0.57
8–11	190	0.45 ± 0.04	0.39	0.40	0.43	0.45	0.48	0.51	0.53
9–12	190	0.43 ± 0.04	0.36	0.38	0.40	0.43	0.45	0.48	0.51
10–13	190	0.41 ± 0.04	0.34	0.36	0.38	0.41	0.43	0.46	0.49
11–14	190	0.39 ± 0.04	0.33	0.34	0.36	0.39	0.41	0.44	0.47
12–15	190	0.37 ± 0.04	0.31	0.32	0.35	0.37	0.39	0.43	0.45
13–16	190	0.36 ± 0.04	0.30	0.31	0.33	0.36	0.38	0.41	0.44
14–17	190	0.35 ± 0.04	0.28	0.30	0.32	0.34	0.37	0.40	0.42
15–18	190	0.33 ± 0.04	0.27	0.28	0.31	0.33	0.35	0.39	0.41
16–19	190	0.32 ± 0.04	0.26	0.27	0.30	0.32	0.34	0.38	0.40
17–20	190	0.31 ± 0.04	0.25	0.26	0.29	0.31	0.33	0.37	0.39
18–21	190	0.03 ± 0.04	0.24	0.25	0.28	0.30	0.32	0.36	0.38
19–22	190	0.03 ± 0.04	0.23	0.25	0.27	0.29	0.31	0.35	0.37
20–23	190	0.29 ± 0.04	0.23	0.24	0.27	0.28	0.31	0.34	0.36
21–24	190	0.28 ± 0.04	0.22	0.23	0.26	0.28	0.30	0.33	0.35

Age (month)	N	Length (mm/day)	Percentile						
			5th	10th	25th	50th	75th	90th	95th
Girls									
Up to 3	562	0.99 ± 0.10	0.82	0.86	0.93	0.99	1.06	1.11	
1–4	74	0.95 ± 0.10	–	0.84	0.87	0.95	1.02	1.07	
2–5	74	0.80 ± 0.10	–	0.67	0.73	0.81	0.87	0.92	
3–6	241	0.67 ± 0.08	0.55	0.58	0.63	0.67	0.72	0.77	
4–7	167	0.60 ± 0.06	0.53	0.54	0.57	0.61	0.64	0.67	
5–8	167	0.56 ± 0.05	0.49	0.50	0.52	0.56	0.59	0.62	
6–9	167	0.52 ± 0.05	0.45	0.46	0.48	0.52	0.55	0.57	
7–10	167	0.48 ± 0.04	0.42	0.43	0.45	0.49	0.52	0.54	
8–11	167	0.46 ± 0.04	0.39	0.41	0.43	0.46	0.49	0.51	
9–12	167	0.44 ± 0.04	0.37	0.38	0.41	0.44	0.46	0.48	
10–13	167	0.42 ± 0.04	0.35	0.37	0.39	0.42	0.45	0.46	
11–14	167	0.40 ± 0.04	0.34	0.35	0.37	0.40	0.43	0.44	
12–15	167	0.38 ± 0.04	0.32	0.34	0.36	0.38	0.41	0.43	
13–16	167	0.37 ± 0.04	0.31	0.32	0.34	0.37	0.40	0.42	
14–17	167	0.36 ± 0.04	0.29	0.31	0.33	0.36	0.38	0.40	
15–18	167	0.34 ± 0.04	0.28	0.30	0.32	0.35	0.37	0.39	0.40
16–19	167	0.33 ± 0.04	0.27	0.29	0.31	0.34	0.36	0.38	0.39
17–20	167	0.32 ± 0.04	0.26	0.28	0.30	0.33	0.35	0.37	0.38
18–21	167	0.32 ± 0.04	0.26	0.27	0.29	0.32	0.34	0.36	0.37
19–22	167	0.31 ± 0.04	0.25	0.26	0.28	0.31	0.33	0.35	0.36
20–23	167	0.30 ± 0.04	0.24	0.26	0.28	0.30	0.33	0.35	0.36
21–24	167	0.29 ± 0.04	0.23	0.25	0.27	0.30	0.32	0.34	0.35

Chapter 2
General Pediatrics

Pediatric Nutrition Handbook: An Algorithmic Approach, First Edition. Edited by David L. Suskind and Polly Lenssen.
© 2011 Blackwell Publishing Ltd. Published 2011 by Blackwell Publishing Ltd.

Nutritional Algorithm for Failure to Thrive (FTT)

Failure to Thrive in Asymptomatic Child

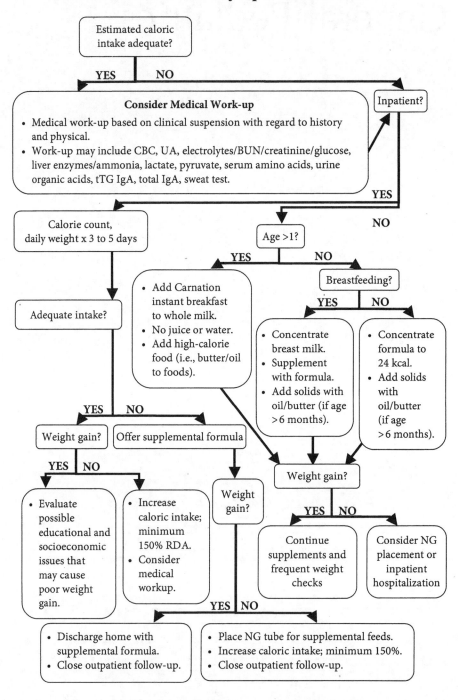

2.1   Failure to Thrive
Crystal Knight, David L. Suskind

2.1.1   Name of Disorder

Failure to thrive (FTT).

2.1.2   Clinical Definition

Inadequate growth, weight gain, or weight for height.

2.1.3   How It Is Diagnosed

Weight for age <3rd percentile or crossing over 2 percentile lines on the growth chart or <80% of ideal body weight for age.

2.1.4   Nutritional Implications

Poor weight gain in childhood is often secondary to poor caloric intake. Long term, this can lead to cognitive defects and stunting.

2.1.5   Pearls

- It is important to distinguish between FTT caused by disease states such as celiac or renal tubular acidosis and FTT caused by poor caloric intake.
- Workup should be guided by physical examination findings as well as medical history.
- Most outpatient FTT in an asymptomatic child is secondary to poor caloric intake as a result of food refusal or excessive juice/water intake.

Nutritional Algorithm for Failure to Gain Weight Breast-Feeding

Failure To Gain Weight Breast-feeding

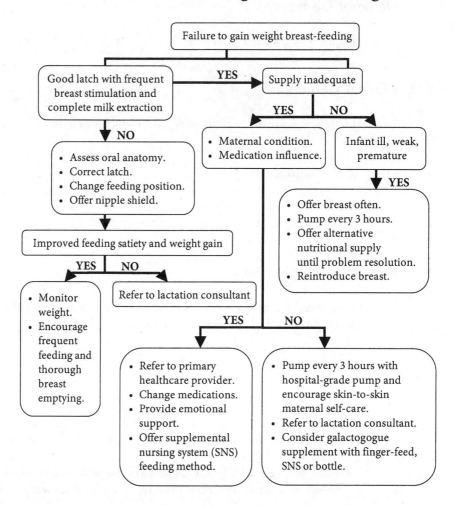

2.2   Failure to Gain Weight Breast-Feeding

Lee Bossung Sweeney

2.2.1   Name of Disorder

Failure to gain weight Breast-Feeding.

2.2.2   How It Is Diagnosed

Weight loss, lethargy, fussiness, low urine and stool output, and lack of satiety after feeding.

2.2.3   Nutritional Implications

Factors that interfere with successful breast-feeding include maternal health, maternal medications, health of infant, frequency of breast stimulation, poor sucking, and incomplete extraction of milk from breasts.

2.2.4   Pearls

- Supplementing with a bottle (and thus infrequent breast stimulation) is the most common cause of loss of milk supply.
- Infant oral motor disorders and maternal condition are rare causes of failure to gain weight but must be considered as part of evaluation.
- Proper latch, frequent suckling, and complete breast emptying are keys to successful breast-feeding.
- Bottle supplementation of healthy mothers and newborns is most often due to lack of confidence in mothering skills, lack of knowledge, and lack of support.

In 2005 the American Academy of Pediatrics (AAP) published its revised policy statement on breast-feeding. In it, the AAP supports exclusive breast-feeding for healthy infants and provides recommendations for physicians and other health care professionals. To support new parents, we must first understand the lactating breast and the important role the infant plays in this mother–infant dance.

2.2.5   Overview of Lactation

Lactogenesis is the process by which the mammary gland develops the capacity to secrete milk. The process begins midpregnancy and continues after delivery with the onset of milk secretion (lactation). After delivery of the placenta, progesterone levels fall quickly, allowing for a rapid onset of milk secretion within 30 to 40 hours of delivery (engorgement). This phase is independent of milk removal. **However, ongoing successful milk production is highly dependent on continual and effective milk removal as defined by frequency, duration, and efficiency of infant suckling and/or maternal expression/pumping.** Suckling stimulates the anterior pituitary gland to secrete prolactin, which triggers breast alveoli to secrete milk and the posterior pituitary gland to secrete oxytocin. In turn, this stimulates the breast alveoli to eject milk ("let-down") into the ducts. The breast begins to return to its prepregnant state (involution) when there is mechanical pressure from the distended gland, together with cessation of stimulation of the gland. Milk stasis, together with the whey protein called feedback inhibitor of lactation (FIL), is believed to set up a cascade of actions that down-regulate milk synthesis.

2.2.6 Supply

Adequacy of milk supply is highly dependent on frequency, duration, and effective suckling/expression. Although breast size may vary widely in the lactating woman, milk supply at various points over time is fairly consistent. Small-breasted woman are capable of producing just as adequate volumes of milk for their infant as a large-breasted woman; however, they may have a smaller storage capacity and may need to feed more frequently. The following is a *guideline* for volumes produced.

Type of Milk	Time Range Expected	Quantity
Colostrum	In the first 24–48 hours	10–100 mL/day Average: 30 mL/day
Mature milk	By 36 hours	~50 mL/day
	By 72 hours	500–600 mL/day
	By 3–4 weeks	700–800 mL/day

Breast-feeding is not fully established until 3–4 weeks after delivery. Introducing alternative feeding methods such as a *bottle for convenience only undermines supply*. The number of times an infant feeds in 24 hours depends on a number of factors, but in the early days to weeks of life, feeding 10 to 12×/day is not uncommon. True inadequate supply in a healthy newborn is not as common as a perceived inadequate supply. This happens when the parents misinterpret the infant's cues of short sleep times, fussiness, and frequent feedings as a sign that the mother is not producing enough milk, and thus parents supplement with cow's milk. Discussing feeding frequency of a breast-versus-formula-fed infant, satiety after feeds, stool and urine output, nutritive versus nonnutritive sucking needs, and weight gain can give parents the tools to assess their infant adequately and boost their confidence as new parents.

- *Galactagogues* are drugs/supplements that may have some effect on increasing milk supply. The most common of these are metoclopramide and domperidone. Their antidopaminergic effect is thought to elevate the release of prolactin and increase milk synthesis. Domperidone has been linked to arrhythmias and is not easily available in the United States for this off-label use. The off-label use of metoclopramide must be used with caution due to the potential side effects of depression and the extrapyramidal symptoms.
- Women take many herbal supplements to increase milk synthesis, the most common of which is *fenugreek*. Although it is frequently used and many women report an increase in milk synthesis, very little evidence or science supports its use. Reported side effects with its use are hypoglycemia (contraindicated in women with diabetes, asthma, or peanut allergies), and it may make the woman's and baby's urine smell like maple syrup.

- Methods to supplement breast-feeding usually involve a bottle. If a bottle must be used and the goal is eventual breast-feeding, then a bottle with a *slow-flow nipple* should be chosen. This provides infants with a similar experience at the breast in that they must suck to extract or transfer the milk. Many nipples simply allow the milk to drip out into the infants' mouths, and all that infants then need to do is to swallow what is in their mouths.
- A *supplemental nursing system (SNS)* is a commercially available unit that is another option to mothers with low milk supply. It promotes suckling (thus increasing milk synthesis) while providing the infant with milk from the breast and supplementation at the same time. A bottle of milk with two small tubes is placed on the mother. The tubes are taped to her breasts. The infant is latched to both the tube and the breast, receiving what is in the mother's breasts and the supplement in the bottle. It also provides breast stimulation to increase milk synthesis.
- *Finger feeding* is a method to administer milk orally to an infant without the use of a bottle. Finger feeding involves taping a small 5 or 6F feeding tube to a parent's finger. Connected to the feeding tube is a syringe full of milk (10 cc is best). As the parent allows the infant to suck on their finger, milk is slowly administered from the syringe as the infant sucks.
- Another method used in some nurseries is cup feeding, in which infants are presented with a small medicine cup of milk and allowed to "lap" it up into their mouths. This method can often waste milk and makes quantifying intake difficult.

2.2.7 Latch and Suck

The goal of latching onto the breast is adequate milk removal or "milk transfer." Simply having the mouth to the nipple is inadequate for milk transfer. Frequent suckling is good to increase volume, but suckling without milk transfer will not increase supply. Therefore, it is imperative to success that adequate latching, sucking, and milk transfer be evaluated.

1. **Proper alignment:** In a *cradle* hold, the infant is flexed and relaxed, with its trunk facing the mother's stomach and its head squarely facing the breast and body and at breast level. The nipple is pointing up toward the baby's nose, and the mother is holding her breast with her fingers in the form of a "C." The mother is relaxed and supported with pillows and a footstool. The *football* hold, in which an infant is lying supine on a pillow, is often preferred for mothers who have had a cesarean delivery or for premature infants. The mother can better visualize her tiny infant's mouth during latch-on in this hold, and for a cesarean delivery mother, there is no pressure on her abdomen.
2. **Areolar grasp:** This is characterized by the infant's gaping, wide-open mouth, with lips flanged outward and the latch covering the nipple and a good bit of areolar tissue. The infant's tongue is troughed, the nipple is on top of the

tongue, and the tongue can extend beyond the alveolar ridge (first rule out ankyloglossia). Infants, especially premature infants whose mothers have extremely large nipples, may have difficulty getting all of the nipple in the mouth, let alone a couple of centimeters of alveolar tissue.

3. **Areolar compression:** The infant's mandible moves rhythmically, gliding back and forth, not in an up-and-down chewing motion, with cheeks remaining full and rounded, not dimpling.

4. **Audible swallowing:** Hard to hear in the first few days as the volume is small; may see three to four sucks prior to swallow in the first few days, and may be heard more frequently after let-down occurs.

Milk transfer can often be assessed by observing the change in the baby's sucking rhythm. Initially, after latching, the baby "flutter-sucks." These are short sucks without swallowing that stimulate the mother's let-down reflex. Once let-down has occurred, the infant's sucking pattern should switch to long, rhythmic draws as milk is transferred and swallowing occurs. Flutter-sucking throughout a feeding indicates there is no milk being transferred, and although infants appear to be suckling, they will usually cry if removed from the breast and act as if they are still hungry (which they are).

Clinical Symptoms of a Poor/Incorrect Latch

Symptoms include pain throughout the feed (not transient discomfort), chomping or biting sensation, smacking or clicking sounds heard, observation of only rapid or flutter sucking, baby falls asleep right away or cries and never seems satiated.

Solutions

Break the suction, evaluate and change the feeding position (the football hold offers the best visualization of latch), make sure the lips are flanged outward, re-latch, perform a digital assessment of latch and trough of tongue, rule out ankyloglossia, consider maternal Candida or bacterial infection if nipples have skin breakdown, and consider evaluation by lactation consultant or infant feeding therapist.

Supplies That Help

- Nipple shield (most often used for short, flat, or inverted nipples or extremely sore nipples). Good for mother/baby struggling with latch.
- Soothies (hydrogel pads) are soothing gel pads for skin breakdown on nipples.
- Sterilized lanolin such as Lansinoh or a few drops of expressed breast milk on nipples for healing.

These items are available in the hospital and at maternity stores in the community.

2.2.8 Lactation and Maternal Medications

The clinician is often faced with questions regarding the safety of mother's breast milk when the mother is taking prescription or over-the-counter medication or undergoing a procedure, nuclear medicine scan, or day surgery. In most cases, breast-feeding does *not* need to be stopped and rarely does the mother have to "pump and dump." A wonderful resource for health care providers regarding lactation and maternal medications is Thomas W. Hale's *Medications and Mother's Milk*. This book provides the clinician with a very comprehensive resource based on the drug's half-life, molecular weight, milk-to-plasma ratios, protein binding, and more. It then delivers a score to each drug based on safety or lactation risk.

2.2.9 Pearls

- Primary failure of lactogenesis can be due to many maternal factors, including type 1 diabetes, maternal obesity, retained placental fragments, polycystic ovarian syndrome, nonelective cesarian delivery, Sheehan syndrome or postpartum hemorrhage, failure to develop adequate mammary glandular tissue, breast reductions (more so than breast augmentation), and some medications.
- Additional factors that negatively influence successful lactation include maternal stress, fatigue, poor breast development (due to delivery prematurely), maternal infant separation, and inadequate frequency of pumping/suckling.
- Inadequate supply does exist, however, regardless of how it evolved. Hospitalized sick infants who cannot go to breast, mothers separated from their infants, stress and lack of access to pump as often as needed are all contributors to a less-than-adequate supply. Solutions include:
- Pumping every 3 hours 8×/day with a properly fitted, double electric, hospital-grade breast pump.
- Breast massage.
- Skin-to-skin time with her infant.
- Self-care (adequate food, fluids, pain management, and rest).
- Routine follow-up with a lactation consultant.
- Breast pumps for purchase in the community are often only satisfactory to maintain an already established milk supply or for only the occasional need to pump when away from the baby.
- Milk synthesis is largely determined by sensitive and active lactocytes, so it is reasonable to conclude that the best indicator of milk synthesis is adequate lactational breast tissue with enlargement of the breasts during pregnancy.

- Supplementing with a bottle is the most common cause of loss of milk supply.
- Infant oral motor disorders and maternal condition are rare causes of infant failure to gain weight, but they must be considered as part of evaluation.
- Proper latching, frequent suckling, and complete breast emptying are the keys to successful breast-feeding.
- Bottle supplementation of healthy mothers and newborns is most often due to lack of confidence in mothering skills, lack of knowledge, and lack of support.

References

American Academy of Pediatrics. Breastfeeding and the use of human milk: policy statement. *Pediatrics*. 2005;115(2):496–506.

Biancuzzo M. *Breastfeeding the Newborn: Clinical Strategies for Nurses*. St. Louis, MO: Mosby; 2003.

Hale TW. *Medications and Mother's Milk*. Amarillo, TX: Hale Publishing; 2008.

Hale TW, Hartmann PE, eds. *Hale & Hartmann's Textbook of Human Lactation*. 13th ed. Amarillo, TX: Hale Publishing; 2007.

Martens PJ, Romphf L. Factors associated with newborn in-hospital weight loss: comparisons by feeding method, demographics and birthing process. *J Hum Lact*. 2007;23(3):233–241.

Nutritional Algorithm for Swallowing Disorder and Aspiration

Swallowing Disorder and Aspiration

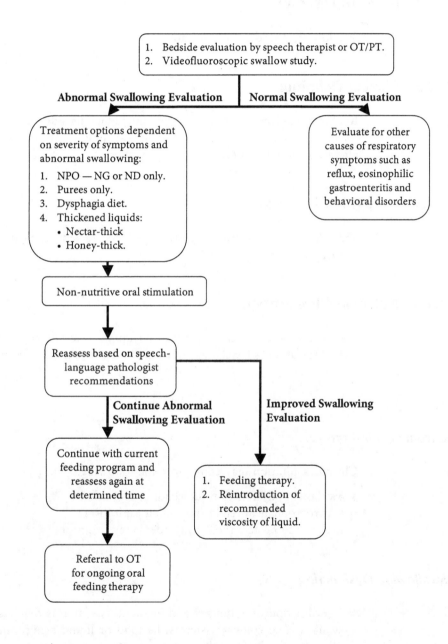

2.3   Swallowing Disorder and Aspiration
Susan Casey

2.3.1   Name of Disorder

Swallowing disorder and aspiration.

2.3.2   Clinical Definition

Repeated passage of food material (including liquids such as breast milk, formula, water, and juice), gastric juices, and/or saliva into the subglottic airways, causing chronic respiratory symptoms.

2.3.3   How It Is Diagnosed

Videofluoroscopic swallowing study (VFSS), bedside clinical evaluation, pH probe, chest x-ray.

2.3.4   Nutritional Implications

Possibility of viscosity change in allowed liquids. Possibility of nothing per mouth (NPO) status. Possible change in the method of feeding liquids and solids.

2.3.5   Pearls

Chronic Aspiration

Chronic aspiration may come from the following:

- Swallowing dysfunction (descending aspiration).
- Gastroesophageal reflux (ascending aspiration).
- Inability to protect the airway adequately from oral secretions.

Swallowing Dysfunction

- Coordination of voluntary and involuntary action is required for a normal swallow. The voluntary step is the food or liquid being transported to the pharynx after it enters the mouth. The involuntary step occurs when the soft palate seals the nasopharynx, and the larynx is elevated and vocal cords close. The pharyngeal constrictors contract, forcing the food or liquid into the esophagus. **Any abnormality in either the voluntary or involuntary process can contribute to subglottic penetration or frank aspiration.**

Aspiration may be silent with the child having no cough or reaction to the food or liquid entering the lungs.

Gastroesophageal Reflux/Ascending Aspiration

- It is possible in an infant or child with gastroesophageal reflux (GER) to introduce acid into the lungs. Acid reflux can cause desquamation of the mucosa, damage to the alveoli, and neutrophilic inflammation.

Descending Aspiration

There are two primary means to identify descending aspiration in infants and children. The VFSS involves contrast added to various viscosities of liquids as well as different textures of foods (depending on the age of the child). A speech-language pathologist (SLP) performs the study in the Radiology Department. All steps in the swallowing process can be seen. A bedside clinical evaluation by a clinician (SLP or occupational therapist/physical therapist) assists in evaluating oral-motor skills but cannot actually visualize or detect aspiration. Dysphagia is often suspected by a clinician, which then needs to followed up by a VFSS.

The VFSS determines what viscosity of liquid is safe or whether or not any liquid *is* safe, in which case the child is made NPO for liquids or whatever food is aspirated. The SLP makes recommendations to the multidisciplinary team managing the child.

Changing Viscosities

Three primary types of products are used to increase the thickness of liquids and prevent descending aspiration:

- **Infant rice cereal:** 1 Tbsp per 2 oz of liquid (nectar thickness), 1 Tbsp per 1 oz liquid (honey thickness).
- **Pros:** Less costly, readily available (such as through Women, Infants and Children). Use requires alteration of the nipple or purchase of a special nipple that allows the thickened liquid to flow.
- **Cons:** Increase in caloric density (1 Tbsp/2 oz adds 7 calories per ounce), which can be problematic in a normal weight or overweight infant or child.
- **Cornstarch-based powdered thickeners:** Guidelines on the container are for adults not pediatric patients. Seattle Children's provides specific guidelines for nectar-thick and honey-thick liquids.
- **Pros:** Less caloric density than rice cereal (1 Tbsp/4 oz adds 4 calories per ounce).
- **Cons:** Cornstarch-based thickeners continue to thicken with time, making a product too thick if it stands too long. Cost can quadruple the cost of rice cereal. Breast milk is difficult to thicken with this type of product. Not always covered by insurance.

- **Gel-based thickeners (xanthan gum):** These thickeners are intended to thicken either to nectar or honey thickness. They are ready to use directly into the liquid.
- **Pros:** Contribute no calories to liquids; do not thicken over time. Best for breast milk.
- **Cons:** Expensive; not always covered by insurance. *Use for infants and children on a ketogenic diet or who are allergic to corn products. Xanthan gums should not be used for premature infants.*

Changing Textures

Based on either clinical evaluation or VFSS, changes in textures of solids foods may be recommended. Various forms of the dysphagia diet may be recommended.

References

Boesch RP, Daines C, Willging JP, et al. Advances in the diagnosis and management of chronic pulmonary aspiration in children. *Eur Respir J.* 2008;28(4):847–861.

Nutritional Algorithm for Gastroesophageal Reflux Disease (GERD)

Gastroesophageal Reflux Disease

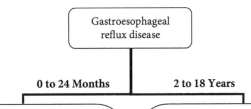

Gastroesophageal reflux disease

0 to 24 Months

- Avoid overfeeding.
- For formula-fed infants, feedings can be thickened by 1 Tbsp of rice cereal per 1 ounce formula (bottle nipple may need to be adjusted).
- May trial hypoallergenic formula.
- Keep infants up for at least 30 minutes after meals.
- Avoid car seat positioning in home.
- Avoid tight diapers/elastic waistbands.
- Avoid smoke exposure.

2 to 18 Years

- Smaller meals more often.
- Avoid eating 2 to 3 hours before bedtime.
- Elevate head off bed 30°.
- Avoid carbonated drinks, chocolate, foods high in fat (e.g., pizza, french fries) or contain a lot of acids (citrus, pickles, tomato products) or spicy foods.
- Avoid large meals with exercise.
- Avoid tobacco smoke exposure and alcohol exposure.

2.4 Gastroesophageal Reflux Disease

David L. Suskind

2.4.1 Name of Disorder

Gastroesophageal reflux disease (GERD).

2.4.2 Clinical Definition

Reflux of gastric contents into the esophagus causing either clinical symptoms or histologic changes on biopsy.

2.4.3 How It Is Diagnosed

During infancy, history may include regurgitation, difficulty eating, fussiness/pain, poor weight gain or weight loss, and recurrent respiratory infections. In older children, symptoms may include heartburn, dysphagia, odynophagia, recurrent respiratory infections, and poor appetite. Clinical diagnosis can be aided by pH probe and endoscopy.

2.4.4   Nutritional Implications

Potential cause of poor growth and feeding aversion in infants and toddlers.

2.4.5   Pearls

- Everyone refluxes; it is only a disease/problem if a patient has a symptom related to reflux (poor weight gain, respiratory symptoms, or pain), or if there are histologic changes to the esophagus.
- Worrisome symptoms that require workup include bilious/blood-tinged emesis, dysphagia, food refusal, breathing difficulty, and odynophagia.
- Fundoplications should be avoided if possible in children <1 year of age and neurologically impaired.

Nutritional Algorithm for Acute Gastroenteritis (AGE)

Acute Gastroenteritis (AGE)

**Vomiting and Diarrhea in Otherwise
Healthy Child Without Comorbid Conditions**

- Greater than 2 months of age.
- Vomit is nonbloody, nonbilious.
- Diarrhea is nonbloody.
- Duration <7 days.

Assess degree of dehydration; routine labs not useful
except in severe dehydration; glucose recommended
if signs and symptoms of hypoglycemia present

Frequent small feedings (every 10 minutes)
of oral rehydration solution (ORS)
or any tolerated foods

Regular/No Dehydration

**Continued Child's Preferred
Age-Appropriate Diet**

- Avoid restrictive diets.
- May add high-pectin foods,
  such as bananas, rice, apples
  and toast, to usual diet.

Mild/Moderate/Severe Dehydration

Oral rehydration
solution (ORS)

Severe dehydration, or if unable
to replace the EFD and keep up
with oral loss using ORS, then:

IVF or NG ORS

Begin refeeding of
usual diet at earliest opportunity
when rehydration is achieved

2.5   Acute Gastroenteritis

David L. Suskind

2.5.1   Name of Disorder

Acute gastroenteritis (AGE).

2.5.2   Clinical Definition

Vomiting and diarrhea in an otherwise healthy child.

2.5.3   How It Is Diagnosed

History and physical.

2.5.4   Nutritional Implications

AGE worldwide is the second leading cause of mortality in pediatrics. Oral rehydration solution (ORS) has played an important role in decreasing morbidity and mortality caused by AGE.

2.5.5   Pearls

- Initial assessment of dehydration in young children should focus on weight loss, general appearance, capillary refill time, skin turgor, and respiratory pattern.
- Routine laboratory tests such as electrolytes and stool studies are not indicated in routine management of AGE. Testing may be useful in children with severe dehydration. Repeat electrolytes may be useful in severe hypernatremia, hyponatremia, hyperkalemia, and hypokalemia.
- Avoid using vague strategies (e.g., IV and PO for rehydration).
- Discharge goal for AGE for patients hospitalized for ≤23 hours should be based on sufficient rehydration not requiring an IV or nasogastric tube, tolerance for ORS, and medical follow-up.
- ORS recipe: Most ORS packets dissolve in 1 L of water to produce a solution containing (in Mmol/L) Na 90, K 20, Cl 8, citrate 10, and glucose 11. Pedialyte can be a safe, ready-made form of ORS.

Based on Seattle Children's Hospital management of acute gastroenteritis by Joel S. Tieder, MD.

Nutritional Algorithm for Cow Milk Protein Allergy

Cow Milk Protein Allergy (CMP)

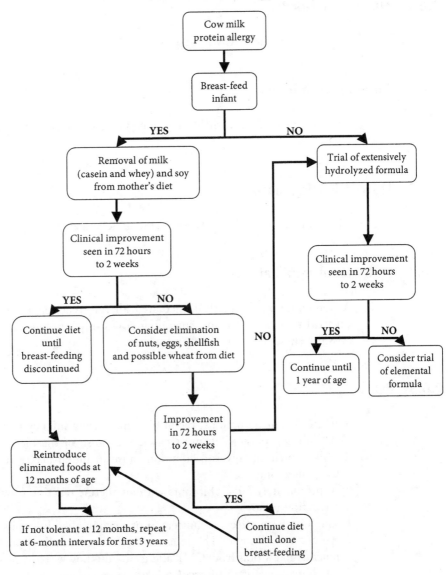

2.6 Cow's Milk Protein Allergy
David L. Suskind

2.6.1 Name of Disorder

Cow's milk protein (CMP) allergy.

2.6.2 Clinical Definition

Disorder of infancy with bloody, mucous-like stools in an otherwise healthy child.

2.6.3 How It Is Diagnosed

Clinical history and physical or histologic changes on biopsy.

2.6.4 Nutritional Implications

A nonimmunoglobulin (Ig)E-mediated allergic reaction in colon and rectum caused by dietary proteins, including cow's milk protein and soy, as well as possibly eggs, shellfish, nuts, and wheat.

2.6.5 Pearls

- In industrialized nations, rectal bleeding during infancy is usually a benign, self-limiting process. In most cases, the cause of the bleeding is unknown. Milk protein allergy is a common cause of blood per rectum in infancy in the United States.
- Approximately 50% of infants with an allergic reaction to whey/casein have a reaction to soy.
- The long-term effects of untreated or uncontrolled low milk-protein allergy are not fully known. The long-term effects of small amounts of bloody or mucous-like stools from CMP allergy are unknown. Therapy should be based on clinical severity and pros/cons of treatments.

Nutritional Algorithm for Eosinophilic Esophagitis

Eosinophilic Esophagitis

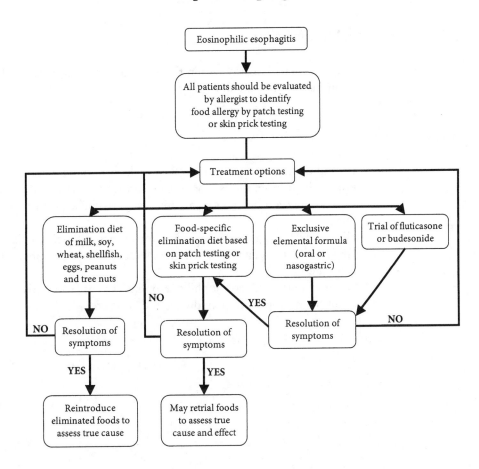

2.7 Eosinophilic Esophagitis

David L. Suskind

2.7.1 Name of Disorder

Eosinophilic esophagitis.

2.7.2 Clinical Definition

Non-IgE-mediated allergy more common in children >1 year of age; present with dysphagia, abdominal pain, vomiting, and/or FTT.

2.7.3   How It Is Diagnosed

Endoscopy with biopsy; biopsy shows increased eosinophils.

2.7.4   Nutritional Implications

Non-IgE-mediated allergy within the esophagus primarily caused by food allergies but also environmental allergies.

2.7.5   Pearls

- IgE radioallergosorbent testing (RAST) does not have a good clinical correlation with eosinophilic esophagitis (a non-IgE-mediated process).
- Most common food allergies are milk, soy, peanuts, shellfish, wheat, and tree nuts.
- Histologic findings on biopsy are sometimes difficult to distinguish from GERD. Therefore, a trial of acid blockade may be warranted if the diagnosis is in question.
- Chronic untreated eosinophilic esophagitis can cause tissue remodeling, resulting in esophageal narrowing and stricture.

Nutritional Algorithm for Food Allergies

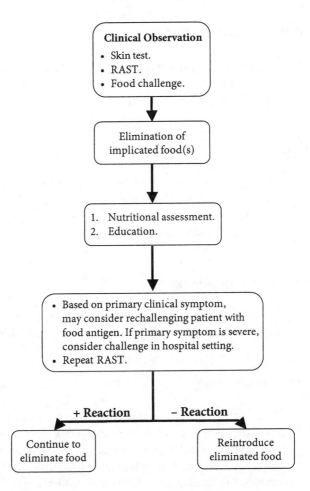

Food Allergies

Clinical Observation
- Skin test.
- RAST.
- Food challenge.

↓

Elimination of implicated food(s)

↓

1. Nutritional assessment.
2. Education.

↓

- Based on primary clinical symptom, may consider rechallenging patient with food antigen. If primary symptom is severe, consider challenge in hospital setting.
- Repeat RAST.

+ Reaction   **– Reaction**

Continue to eliminate food   Reintroduce eliminated food

2.8   Food Allergies
Susan Casey

2.8.1   Name of Disorder

Food allergies.

2.8.2   Clinical Definition

An immunologically mediated adverse reaction to proteins within foods. The major immunologic components are eosinophils mast cells, basophils, and IgE.

2.8.3   How It Is Diagnosed

Clinical observation, skin testing, RAST, and food challenge.

2.8.4   Nutritional Implications

Dietary restrictions can lead to an unbalanced diet and poor growth. Serious life-threatening events can result from intentional or inadvertent ingestion of food-causing allergic reaction.

2.8.5   Pearls

True food allergies are IgE mediated. There are other conditions that require elimination of food that are not IgE mediated. *Food intolerance* is not a true food allergy but an abnormal response to a food or food additive (e.g., lactose intolerance and fructose intolerance).

The Most Common Food Allergies

The most common food allergies in pediatric patients are cow milk, egg, peanut, soybean products, fin fish, shellfish, corn, and wheat.

Less Common Food Allergies

Tree nuts, citrus fruits, tomato products, and "latex-related" foods. Children who are allergic to natural rubber latex may have allergic reactions to foods that contain similar components to the protein in latex. Foods with a high degree of association are bananas, avocados, and chestnuts. Other fruits, vegetables, and grains have a lower or undetermined association with latex.

Some food allergies can be correlated to allergies to pollen:

- Mugwort: Carrot, celery, apple, peanut, kiwi.
- Birch: Apple, pear, peach, cherry, hazelnut.
- Grasses: Potato.
- Ragweed: Banana, melon.

These allergies may produce oral allergy syndrome.

Common Allergic Reactions

Asthma, hives, stomach cramps, diarrhea, vomiting, and anaphylaxis. (These reactions can also be indicative of other conditions.)

Food Labeling

The federal Food Allergen Labeling and Consumer Protection Act of 2004 is designed to protect children from ingesting an allergen inadvertently. Food labeling language is required to list foods by their common names. It also requires a manufacturer to list foods that are processed in the same plant (cow milk, egg, fin fish, shellfish, tree nuts, wheat, peanuts, and soybeans). This applies to foods manufactured in the United States.

Common Obstacles

Lack of compliance is one the most common causes of relapse. Lack of compliance is caused most often by lack of knowledge, two households with differing management techniques, denial ("My child doesn't really have an allergy"), and language and culture barriers.

School lunch programs, day-care centers, other households involved, and the school nurse need to be notified of any required allergens to be eliminated.

Patient and Family Education

Patient education materials for individual foods to be eliminated need to include foods to check for on a label, foods to avoid, foods allowed, a sample menu for the day, and resources for the family locally and online.

A nutritional assessment at the time of the education session is an important way to determine if children are at risk for malnutrition before further restriction of their diets. Sharing this information with the primary care provider is important. Sequential visits should track weight gain and growth with adjustments in caloric intake based on nutritional status.

The Food Allergy and Anaphylaxis Network information should be given to the family for newsletters and other products that may be supportive (www.foodallergy.org).

Outgrowing Food Allergies

About 85% of children with milk and egg allergies outgrow their allergy, and 20% of children with peanut allergies outgrow their allergy (when diagnosed <2 *years of age*). A positive skin test may occur for a long period of time after a child is no longer clinically symptomatic of the food allergy.

References

Metcalfe DD, Sampson HA, Simon RA. *Food Allergy: Adverse Reactions to Foods and Food Additives.* 2nd ed. Malden, MA: Blackwell Science; 1997.

Nutritional Algorithm for Toddler's Diarrhea

Toddler's Diarrhea

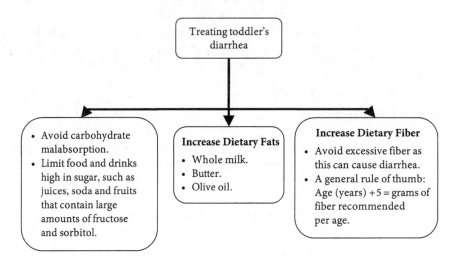

Treating toddler's diarrhea

- Avoid carbohydrate malabsorption.
- Limit food and drinks high in sugar, such as juices, soda and fruits that contain large amounts of fructose and sorbitol.

Increase Dietary Fats
- Whole milk.
- Butter.
- Olive oil.

Increase Dietary Fiber
- Avoid excessive fiber as this can cause diarrhea.
- A general rule of thumb: Age (years) + 5 = grams of fiber recommended per age.

2.9   Toddler's Diarrhea or Chronic, Nonspecific Diarrhea of Childhood

David L. Suskind

2.9.1   Name of Disorder

Toddler's diarrhea or chronic, nonspecific diarrhea of childhood.

2.9.2   Clinical Definition

Disorder of childhood characterized by multiple large, soft to liquid-type stools per day in an otherwise healthy child.

2.9.3   How It Is Diagnosed

Clinically.

2.9.4   Nutritional Implications

Despite often having undigested food particles in the stool, such as corn, these patients are gaining weight well and have no evidence of poor nutrition.

2.10 **Vitamins and Minerals**
Matt Giefer, David L. Suskind

Vitamin/Mineral	Pearl	Symptoms Associated with Deficiency	Risk Factors for Deficiency	Symptoms Associated with Toxicity	Laboratory Tests Associated with Deficiency
Thiamine (vitamin B₁)	Essential coenzyme in carbohydrate metabolism Denatured at high pH and high temperatures Found in yeast, legumes, pork, and cereals	Beriberi • Dry beriberi: Symmetric peripheral neuropathy • Wet beriberi: Edema, congestive heart failure • Infantile beriberi (breastfed children with mother who have subclinical thiamine deficiency): Hoarse weak cry, vomiting and poor feeding, shock Wernicke encephalopathy: Nystagmus, ophthalmalgia, ataxia, and altered mental status Korsakoff syndrome: Amnesia, confabulation, polyneuritis	Patients with food faddisms, anorexics, gastric bypass surgery, long-term total parenteral nutrition, and chronic use of loop diuretics	No known	Transketolase activation test, erythrocyte thiamine transketolase (ETKA), thiamine pyrophosphate (TPP)

Vitamin/Mineral	Pearl	Symptoms Associated with Deficiency	Risk Factors for Deficiency	Symptoms Associated with Toxicity	Laboratory Tests Associated with Deficiency
Vitamin B_2 (riboflavin)	Precursors of the enzyme cofactors flavin mononucleotide and flavin adenine dinucleotide (FAD) that catalyze several mitochondrial oxidation and reduction reactions and function as electron transporters Found in animal proteins, green vegetables and fortified cereals	Nonspecific symptoms but may include sore throat, pharyngeal hyperemia, cheilitis, angular stomatitis, glossitis (magenta tongue), anemia, and dermatitis	Economically disadvantaged with limited milk and meat, anorexia nervosa, kwashiorkor, prolonged severe malabsorption as in celiac or short gut syndrome	No known	Erythrocyte glutathione reductase activity or 24-hour urine collection for riboflavin concentration
Niacin (vitamin B_3)	Form coenzymes NAD and NADP, which are involved in oxidation-reduction reactions Can be synthesized in liver and kidneys from tryptophan Widely distributed in plant and animal foods including beans and fortified cereals	Pellagra("rough skin"): Photosensitive pigmented dermatitis, diarrhea, dementia, death	Severely malnourished patients, complication of alcoholism, anorexia nervosa, and severe malabsorptive states	Flushing, nausea, vomiting, pruritus, maculopathy, and hepatotoxicity	24-hour urine collection of niacin and its metabolite N1-methylnicotinamide, or erythrocyte NAD and NADP concentration

Vitamin/Mineral	Pearl	Symptoms Associated with Deficiency	Risk Factors for Deficiency	Symptoms Associated with Toxicity	Laboratory Tests Associated with Deficiency
Pyridoxine (vitamin B_6)	Unusual as an isolated nutritional deficiency Acts as a coenzyme in amino acid and carbohydrate metabolism Foods rich in pyridoxine include bananas, fish, milk, yeast, eggs, and fortified cereals	Nonspecific symptoms including glossitis, stomatitis, cheilosis, irritability, and confusion Epileptiform convulsions in infants	Low socioeconomic status, isoniazid therapy, and pyridoxine-dependent syndromes	Peripheral sensory neuropathy characterized by bilateral parasthesia, hyperesthesia, limb pain, and ataxia	Plasma pyridoxal 5'-phosphate (PLP)
Folic acid (vitamin B_9)	Necessary for synthesis of purines and thymin, which are required for DNA synthesis In animal products and leafy vegetables, cereal/grains/bread are fortified with folate in the United States	Megaloblastic anemia, pregnancy complications (neural tube defects), cardiovascular disease, colorectal cancer, dementia	Inadequate intake of folate is not rare in children especially with high-fat and sugar diets Anorexia nervosa, malabsorptive diseases and drug interference (pyrimethamine, methotrexate, phenytoin) may also cause deficiency	No known	Megaloblastic macrocytic anemia Red cell folate, serum homocysteine level, serum methymalonic acid level

Vitamin/Mineral	Pearl	Symptoms Associated with Deficiency	Risk Factors for Deficiency	Symptoms Associated with Toxicity	Laboratory Tests Associated with Deficiency
Cobalamin (vitamin B_{12})	Functions as a coenzyme in red blood cell maturation and central nervous system development Involved in DNA synthesis and regulation Only found in animal-derived foods	Infants: Macrocytic megaloblastic anemia, poor growth, movement disorders, development delay Older children/adults: Macrocytic megaloblastic anemia, decreased appetite, constipation, and neurologic problems such as ataxia, muscle weakness, mood disturbances, and psychosis	In infancy, cobalamin deficiency can occur secondary to maternal deficiency in breast-feeding mothers on a vegan diet In older individuals, may occur in bariatric surgery, malabsorptive states, or with ileal disease/resection	No known	Megaloblastic macrocytic anemia Serum homocysteine level, serum methylmalonic acid level, serum cobalamin level
Vitamin C	Functions in folic acid metabolism, collagen biosynthesis, and iron absorption Dietary sources include citrus fruits, tomatoes, potatoes, strawberries, and cantaloupe	Scurvy: bleeding gums, perifollicular hemorrhage, diarrhea, and can progress to bone pain and arthropathy	Rare but case reports noted in children who ingest only well cooked foods with few fruits or vegetables	Diarrhea, renal oxalate stones, hemolysis, abdominal pain, and gas	Ascorbate concentration in blood leukocytes, plasma ascorbate concentration

Vitamin/Mineral	Pearl	Symptoms Associated with Deficiency	Risk Factors for Deficiency	Symptoms Associated with Toxicity	Laboratory Tests Associated with Deficiency
Vitamin A (retinol and derivatives)	Maintenance of proper vision, epithelial cell integrity, and regulation of glycoprotein synthesis and cell differentiation. Almost exclusively from animal sources. Provitamin A (i.e., carotenoids) are in green/orange vegetables	Nyctalopia, xerophthalmia, bitot spots, keratomalacia, impaired resistance to infection, follicular hyperkeratosis and poor bone growth	Patients with chronic fat malabsorption from either luminal disease or pancreatic insufficiency	Anorexia, vomiting, and headaches (increased intracranial pressure), painful bone lesions, hepatotoxicity, dermatitis, alopecia	Plasma retinol and retinol binding protein, conjunctival impression cytology
Vitamin D (calciferol)	Prohormone essential for bone formation and calcium homeostasis. Two forms: D_2 (obtained in diet from plants and fungi) and D_3 (synthesized in skin from sunlight)	Hypocalcemia, hypophosphatemia, tetany, but often asymptomatic. Rickets and osteomalacia. Physical findings: frontal bossing, craniotabes, rachitic rosary, Harrison groove, enlargement of wrists, bowing of distal radial/ulnar, lateral bowing of femur and tibia	Poor intake, increased BMI, prolonged breastfeeding without vitamin D supplement and avoidance of sun exposure	Hypercalcemia may lead to CNS depression, hypercalciuria and ectopic calcification (nephrocalcinosis and nephrolithiasis)	25-hydroxy vitamin D level, calcium, phosphate, alkaline phosphatase, parathyroid hormone

Vitamin/Mineral	Pearl	Symptoms Associated with Deficiency	Risk Factors for Deficiency	Symptoms Associated with Toxicity	Laboratory Tests Associated with Deficiency
Vitamin E (tocopherol and tocotrienols)	Primarily functions as an antioxidant Food sources include oil-containing grains, plants, and vegetables	Extremely rare unless predisposing medical condition; symptoms of deficiency are progressive neurologic symptoms including ataxia, hyporeflexia, impaired balance, and peripheral neuropathy	Biliary atresia, chronic cholestatic liver disease, pancreatic insufficiency	Pro-oxidant effect	Plasma alpha-tocopherol and ratio of plasma alpha tocopherol to total lipids
Vitamin K (2 methyl-1,4 naphthoquinones)	Necessary for posttranslational carboxylation of glutamic acid residues of vitamin K–dependent coagulation proteins	Hypoprothrombinemia and hemorrhagic disease	Newborn infants not supplemented at birth (breast milk has a low amount of vitamin K, and low bacteria count in the infant intestine leads to low production), older children with pancreatic insufficiency and chronic liver disease	Rare; infants can have hemolytic anemia, hyperbilirubinemia, and kernicterus	Prothrombin time, vitamin K–dependent factors (factors II, VII, IX, X), plasma phylloquinone

Vitamin/Mineral	Pearl	Symptoms Associated with Deficiency	Risk Factors for Deficiency	Symptoms Associated with Toxicity	Laboratory Tests Associated with Deficiency
Copper	Component of metalloenzymes and plays role in connective tissue biosynthesis Found in meats, shellfish, legumes and cheese	Sideroblastic anemia, delayed growth osteopenia, neutropenia	Isolated deficiency very rare but has been reported in burn victims and in cases of short bowel syndrome or after bariatric surgery	Wilson disease, nausea, vomiting, diarrhea, renal dysfunction	Serum copper
Iodine	Involved in production of thyroid hormone Iodized salt, diary products, seafood	Goiter, impaired mental function, developmental delay	Less common in the United States given iodination of salt; smoking reduces iodine in breast milk	Oral numbness/ burning, fever, nausea, vomiting, diarrhea	Thyroid stimulating hormone, free thyroxine
Iron	Most common cause of microcytic nutritional deficiency in children	Microcytic hypochromic anemia, pica and pagophagia, lethargy, irritability, poor feeding, esophageal web, impaired neurodevelopment of infants and children	At or below poverty level, prematurity, low birth weight infants, black/ Hispanic toddlers, obesity, prolonged exclusive breast-feeding, vegetarian/ vegan diet, early introduction of cow's milk	Acute: Nausea, vomiting, abdominal pain, tarry stools, coma, organ failure, death Chronic: Diarrhea, constipation	Red blood cell distribution width (RDW), hemoglobin, serum ferritin, percent total iron binding capacity saturation, mean corpuscular volume, zinc protoporphyrin concentration

Vitamin/Mineral	Pearl	Symptoms Associated with Deficiency	Risk Factors for Deficiency	Symptoms Associated with Toxicity	Laboratory Tests Associated with Deficiency
Selenium	Component of glutathione peroxidase, and deiodinase Found in meats, seafood, whole grains	Cardiomyopathy	Areas with low selenium content in the soil (Keshan and Kashin-Beck disease) In industrialized nations, infants and children with severe dietary restrictions and prolonged parenteral nutrition	Rare; irritability, "garlic breath," brittle hair and nails, fatigue	Serum and red blood cell selenium, glutathione peroxidase activity
Zinc	Cofactor for many enzymes involved in nucleic acid and protein metabolism Founds in meats, liver, cheese, and whole grains	Acro-orificial skin lesions, nyctalopia, diarrhea, anorexia, hypogeusia, delayed growth or sexual maturation, impaired wound healing	Associated with protein energy malnutrition, Crohn's disease, sickle cell anemia, and nephrotic syndrome Mild zinc deficiencies can occur in vegan/vegetarian diets high in phytates	Diarrhea and vomiting May aggravate copper deficiency	Serum zinc (although levels correlate poorly to total body stores)

Kleinman R, ed. *Pediatric Nutrition Handbook.* 6th ed. Elk Grove Village, IL: American Academy of Pediatrics; 2009.
Trace Elements in Human Nutrition and Health. Geneva, Switzerland: World Health Organization; 1996.
Requirements of Vitamin A, Iron, Folate and Vitamin B12. Report of a Joint FAO/WHO Expert Consultation. Rome, Italy: Food and Agriculture Organization of the United Nations, 1988 (FAO Food and Nutrition Series, No. 23).
Vitamin and Mineral Requirements in Human Nutrition. 2nd ed. Rome, Italy: World Health Organization and Food and Agriculture Organization of the United Nations; 2004.

Chapter 3
Endocrine

3.1 Type 1 and Type 2 Diabetes Mellitus
Tran Hang

3.1.1 Name of Disorder

Type 1 and Type 2 diabetes.

3.1.2 Clinical Definition

Type 1 diabetes is an autoimmune disease that causes the body to eventually stop producing the pancreatic hormone insulin. Type 2 diabetes is generally a result of the body becoming resistant to insulin or an inadequate insulin compensatory response.

3.1.3 How It Is Diagnosed

Clinical and laboratory studies showing elevated fasting-, postprandial-, or postglucose tolerance test glucoses. The assessment of C-peptide level and autoantibodies can help distinguish between type 1 and type 2 diabetes.

3.1.4 Nutritional Implications

Children with diabetes follow a meal plan that is less stringent than adults because they need adequate calories, protein, vitamins, and minerals to support adequate growth. Adjusting a child's insulin doses to a healthy, well-balanced

Pediatric Nutrition Handbook: An Algorithmic Approach, First Edition. Edited by David L. Suskind and Polly Lenssen.
© 2011 Blackwell Publishing Ltd. Published 2011 by Blackwell Publishing Ltd.

diet is recommended as opposed to restricting carbohydrates to control blood glucose. Children with type 1 diabetes on a long-acting insulin (i.e., Lantus/Glargine) regimen and short-acting insulin (Humalog or NovoLog) regimen follow a balanced diet with carbohydrate counting. Accurate carbohydrate counting is required to determine how much short-acting insulin a child needs to cover each meal or snack. The amount of bolus insulin is determined by the child's prescribed insulin-to-carbohydrate ratio.

3.1.5   Signs and Symptoms of Elevated Blood Glucose

- Polyuria, polydipsia, polyphagia, weight loss.

Diagnostic Parameters

- Fasting plasma glucose:
- Normal: <100 mg/dL.
- Impaired fasting glucose: 100–125 mg/dL.
- Diabetes: ≥126 mg/dL.
- 2-hour postprandial glucose:
- Normal: <140 mg/dL.
- Impaired glucose tolerance: 140–199 mg/dL.
- Diabetes: ≥200 mg/dL.

Type 1 Diabetes

Elevated blood sugar with low fasting C-peptide/insulin level and positive autoantibodies.

Type 2 Diabetes

Elevated blood sugar with high fasting C-peptide/insulin level without autoantibodies.

3.1.6   Nutrition Guidelines for Type 1 Diabetes

- An appropriate calorie level based on a child's age for maintaining a healthy weight and supporting adequate growth.
- A healthy meal plan that includes daily recommended servings from each food groups.
- A carbohydrate intake of 40–60% of total calorie needs is generally recommended. Parents and caregivers are educated to adjust insulin dose based on an insulin-to-carbohydrate ratio rather than restrict calories or carbohydrates to control blood glucose levels.

- A low glycemia index or glycemic load provides only a modest benefit in controlling postprandial blood.
- Protein intake is 15–20% of total calories.
- Follow heart-healthy guidelines:
- For dyslipidemia: Follow an American Heart Association Therapeutic Lifestyle Changes (TLC) diet.
- Limit saturated fat to <7% of total calories.
- Limit intake of trans fat in the diet.
- Limit dietary cholesterol to <200 mg/day.
- Avoid or limit concentrated sweets such as baked goods, juices, and regular sugared sodas.
- Keep in mind that sugar free is not always carbohydrate free.
- Read food labels carefully; pay attention to serving size, total grams of carbohydrates, and amount of dietary fiber. If dietary fiber is ≥5 g per serving, then subtract the grams of dietary fiber from the grams of total carbohydrate, and the difference is the carbohydrate amount consumed at the meal/snack.
- Eat three meals per day. Snacking is not necessary unless there are more than 4- to 5-hour gaps between main meals or the need to prevent low blood glucose due to intense physical activity or to treat for a low-blood glucose event. Generally, younger children may need three meals and one to three snacks per day, and older children/teens may need three meals and no to one snack per day.
- Check blood glucose minimally four times per day: Before breakfast, before lunch, before dinner, and before bedtime.

3.1.7 Nutrition Guidelines for Type 2 Diabetes

- Maintain a healthy weight for age and height by following a balanced meal plan that includes daily recommended servings from each food group and staying physically active.
- Keep carbohydrate intake to 40–60% of total calorie needs.
- Follow the heart-healthy guidelines.
- Children with dyslipidemia are recommended to improve their blood glucose control and follow an American Heart Association TLC diet.
- Limit saturated fat to <7% of total calories.
- Limit intake of trans fat in the diet.
- Limit dietary cholesterol to <200 mg/day.
- Avoid or limit concentrated sweets such as baked goods, juices, and regular sugared sodas.
- Keep in mind that sugar free is not always carbohydrate free.
- Read food labels carefully; pay attention to serving size, total grams of carbohydrates, and amount of dietary fiber. If dietary fiber is ≥5 g per serving, subtract the grams of dietary fiber from the grams of total carbohydrate, and the difference is the amount you use to estimate how much carbohydrate is consumed at the meal/snack.

- Eat three meals per day. Avoid skipping meals and grazing on snacks throughout the day. Unless you are taking insulin, it is not common to experience low blood glucose even if you are taking oral agents such as Metformin/Glucophage (an insulin sensitizer).
- Check your blood glucose one to three times per day or as prescribed by your health care provider based on your diabetes management and control.
- For individuals who are insulin-resistant solely secondary to obesity, a weight loss of 15–20% of baseline weight can resolve the insulin resistance.

3.1.8 Pearls

- The American Diabetes Association hemoglobin A1c treatment goal:
- <6 years of age: 7.5–8.5%.
- 6–12 years of age: <8%.
- 13–19 years of age: <7.5%.
- 19 years of age: <7%.
- Studies have shown medical nutrition therapy can reduce A1c level by 1–2%.
- Converting A1c percentage to mg/dL blood glucose level:
- A1c 5%: ~100 mg/dL.
- Each 1%: ~35 mg/dL.
- 7% A1c: ~170 mg/dL.

References

American Diabetes Association. Diagnosis and classification of diabetes mellitus. *Diabetes Care.* 2008;31(1 Suppl):S55–S60.

American Diabetes Association. Summary of revisions for the 2008 clinical practice recommendations. *Diabetes Care.* 2008;31(1 Suppl):S3–S4.

Bantle JP, Wylie-Rosett J, Albright A, et al. Nutrition recommendations and interventions for diabetes: a position statement of the American Diabetes Association. *Diabetes Care.* 2008;31(1 Suppl):S61–S78.

Franz, MJ, ed. *A Core Curriculum for Diabetes Education: Diabetes Management Therapies.* 5th ed. Chicago, IL: American Association of Diabetes Educators; 2003.

Chapter 4

Gastroenterology

Nutritional Algorithm for Crohn's Disease

Crohn's Disease

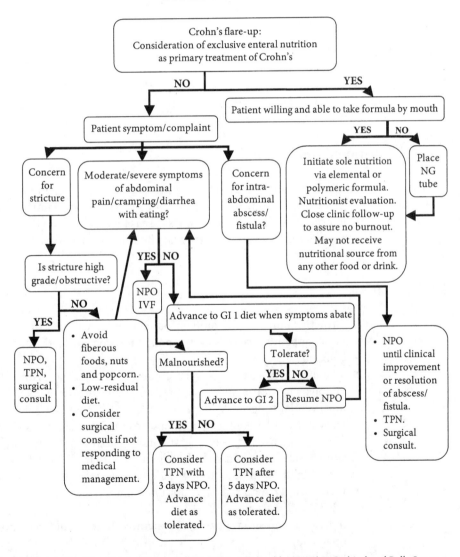

Pediatric Nutrition Handbook: An Algorithmic Approach, First Edition. Edited by David L. Suskind and Polly Lenssen.

4.1   Crohn's Disease
Crystal Knight, David L. Suskind

4.1.1   Name of Disorder

Crohn's disease, regional enteritis.

4.1.2   Clinical Definition

Chronic bowel inflammation secondary to an autoimmune reaction to intestinal tract affecting any region from mouth to anus.

4.1.3   How It Is Diagnosed

History, physical, and gastrointestinal histologic changes in conjunction with laboratory and radiology studies.

4.1.4   Nutritional Implications

Abdominal pain and diarrhea lead to poor oral intake, and inflammation leads to poor absorption, resulting in poor growth. Many nutrient deficiencies are common in patients with Crohn's disease as well. Growth failure is found in 30% of Crohn's disease patients at the time of diagnosis.

4.1.5   Pearls

- Growth failure is common in patients with Crohn's disease, secondary to poor appetite, early satiety, poor absorption, and increased metabolic demand.
- Vitamin D deficiency is very common in children with Crohn's disease. Supplementation is often required to assure proper intake, especially in the northern latitudes.
- Deficiencies of folate, calcium, and iron are quite common in patients with Crohn's disease, as well as fat-soluble vitamins, vitamin B_{12}, magnesium, copper, selenium, and zinc. It is important that all patients be supplemented with a multivitamin as well as calcium and iron if deficient.
- Permanent growth failure is not uncommon in Crohn's disease, occurring in 19–35% of patients.
- Individuals on sulfasalazine and methotrexate should be supplemented with folic acid.
- Individuals who have Crohn's disease who are not in flare-up are recommended to have a regular well-balanced diet without restriction.

Nutritional Algorithm for Ulcerative Colitis

Ulcerative Colitis

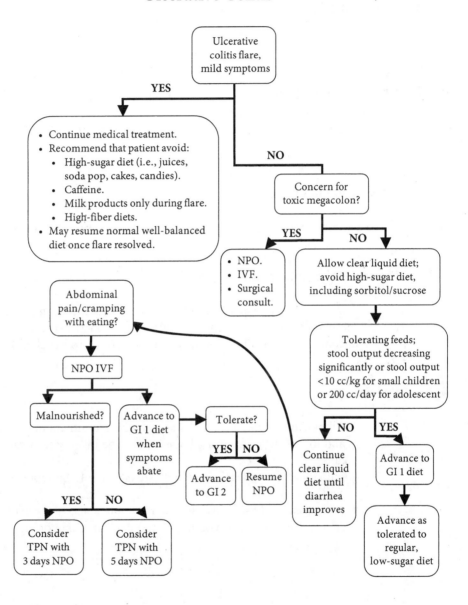

4.2   Ulcerative Colitis

Crystal Knight, David L. Suskind

4.2.1   Name of Disorder

Ulcerative colitis.

4.2.2   Clinical Definition

Chronic bowel inflammation secondary to an autoimmune reaction to the large intestine.

4.2.3   How It Is Diagnosed

History physical histology in conjunction with laboratory and radiology studies.

4.2.4   Nutritional Implications

Although bloody diarrhea can lead to poor oral intake, ulcerative colitis rarely causes nutritional deficiencies apart from iron deficiency. Growth failure is uncommon in ulcerative colitis compared with Crohn's disease.

4.2.5   Pearls

- All patients should be supplemented with a multivitamin, as well as calcium and iron if deficient. Iron should always be taken with vitamin C or orange juice.
- Individuals on sulfasalazine/methotrexate should be supplemented with folic acid.
- Prolonged use of steroids can lead to osteomalacia and osteopenia; therefore, supplementation with vitamin D and calcium is important if deficient.

Nutritional Algorithm for Short Bowel Syndrome

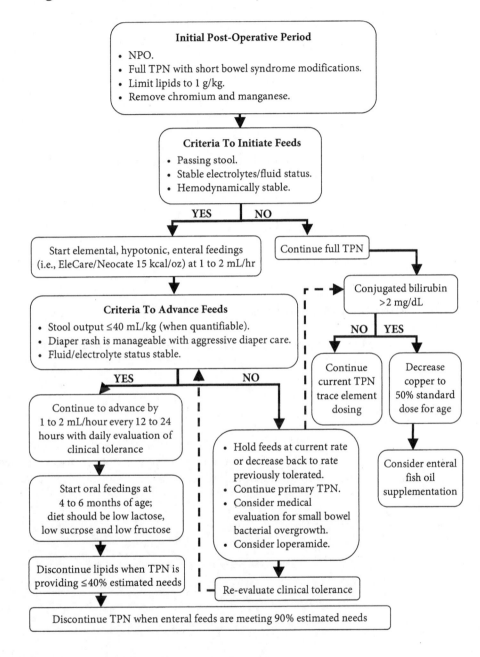

Initial Post-Operative Period
- NPO.
- Full TPN with short bowel syndrome modifications.
- Limit lipids to 1 g/kg.
- Remove chromium and manganese.

Criteria To Initiate Feeds
- Passing stool.
- Stable electrolytes/fluid status.
- Hemodynamically stable.

YES NO

Start elemental, hypotonic, enteral feedings (i.e., EleCare/Neocate 15 kcal/oz) at 1 to 2 mL/hr

Continue full TPN

Conjugated bilirubin >2 mg/dL

NO YES

Criteria To Advance Feeds
- Stool output ≤40 mL/kg (when quantifiable).
- Diaper rash is manageable with aggressive diaper care.
- Fluid/electrolyte status stable.

Continue current TPN trace element dosing

Decrease copper to 50% standard dose for age

YES NO

Continue to advance by 1 to 2 mL/hour every 12 to 24 hours with daily evaluation of clinical tolerance

Consider enteral fish oil supplementation

- Hold feeds at current rate or decrease back to rate previously tolerated.
- Continue primary TPN.
- Consider medical evaluation for small bowel bacterial overgrowth.
- Consider loperamide.

Start oral feedings at 4 to 6 months of age; diet should be low lactose, low sucrose and low fructose

Discontinue lipids when TPN is providing ≤40% estimated needs

Re-evaluate clinical tolerance

Discontinue TPN when enteral feeds are meeting 90% estimated needs

4.3   Short Bowel Syndrome
Cheryl Davis, Simon Horslen

4.3.1   Name of Disorder

Short bowel syndrome or intestinal failure.

4.3.2   Clinical Definition

Malabsorptive state that occurs after significant portion of the small bowel has been resected.

4.3.3   How It Is Diagnosed

Clinical diagnosis based on history and symptoms of malabsorption.

4.3.4   Nutritional Implications

Macronutrient malabsorption, micronutrient malabsorption, and hydration issues.

4.3.5   Pearls

- If patient cannot be weaned off parenteral nutrition by 3 months of age, has significant bowel resection, or shows signs of liver disease, patient should be referred to intestinal failure team.

Nutritional Algorithm for Ascites and Portal Hypertension

Ascites and Portal Hypertension

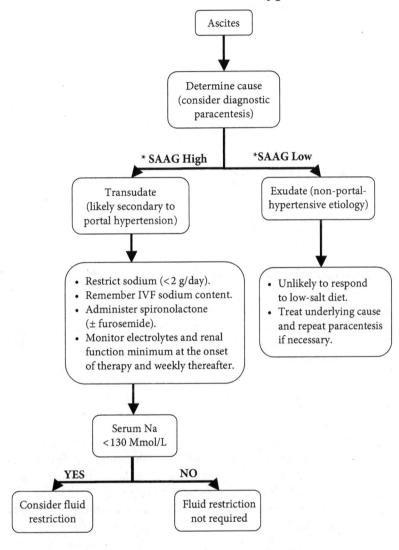

*SAAG = Serum ascites albumin gradient.

4.4   Ascites and Portal Hypertension

Crystal Knight, Simon Horslen

4.4.1   Name of Disorder

Ascites and portal hypertension.

4.4.2   Clinical Definition

Free fluid in the peritoneal cavity.

4.4.3   How It Is Diagnosed

Physical examination (fluid wave, flank bulging, shifting dullness, and "puddle sign") and ultrasonography.

4.4.4   Nutritional Implications

Severe malnutrition with loss of fat stores and muscle wasting affects most children with chronic liver disease, secondary to reduced energy intake, fat malabsorption, disturbed hepatic metabolism, and increased energy expenditure.

4.4.5   Pearls

- Following a patient's nutritional status with ascites can be difficult because the patient's weight reflects both changes in fluid status and true body mass; therefore, other methods such as laboratory investigation and measurement of skinfold thickness may be required.
- Medium-chain triglycerides supplementation may be required because long-chain triglycerides are poorly absorbed.
- Fat-soluble vitamin supplementation is essential.

Nutritional Algorithm for Acute Pancreatitis

Acute Pancreatitis

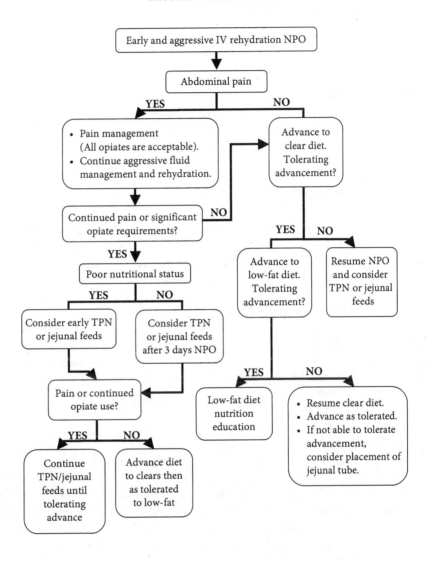

4.5   Acute Pancreatitis

Matt Giefer, Crystal Knight, David L. Suskind

4.5.1   Name of Disorder

Acute pancreatitis.

4.5.2   Clinical Definition

Inappropriate activation of pancreatic digestive enzymes leading to pancreatic/systemic inflammation.

4.5.3   How It Is Diagnosed

Two of the following three elements must be present: abdominal pain, serum lipase levels greater than three times the upper limit of normal, and radiologic evidence of pancreatic inflammation.

4.5.4   Nutritional Implications

Eating may aggravate symptoms during an acute episode, and patients may require parenteral nutrition or enteral feedings distal to the duodenum. Pancreatic exocrine insufficiency and fat malabsorption may develop if sufficient pancreatic tissue is destroyed.

4.5.5   Pearls

- Differential for acute pancreatitis is broad; however, in children most cases of acute pancreatitis are idiopathic or in the setting of multiorgan dysfunction. Other causes of pancreatitis include trauma, metabolic abnormalities, hereditary/familial pancreatitis, medication side effects, viral infection, pancreatic duct obstruction, or anatomic abnormality.
- Initial workup should include a detailed history, including medication review, serum electrolytes with ionized calcium, triglyceride levels, and imaging. If multiple episodes occur, referral to a specialist should be considered.
- Current evidence suggests that early enteral nutrition via nasojejunal feeds improves outcomes for patients with severe acute pancreatitis.
- For children with mild acute pancreatitis, advancing feeds is still a clinical judgment call, with patient's symptomatic improvement of paramount importance. Laboratory indices do not always correlate with symptoms, although laboratory trends can be helpful in clinical decision making.

Chapter 5
Biochemical Genetics

Pediatric Nutrition Handbook: An Algorithmic Approach, First Edition. Edited by David L. Suskind and Polly Lenssen.
© 2011 Blackwell Publishing Ltd. Published 2011 by Blackwell Publishing Ltd.

Nutritional Algorithm for Urea Cycle Defects

Urea Cycle Defects

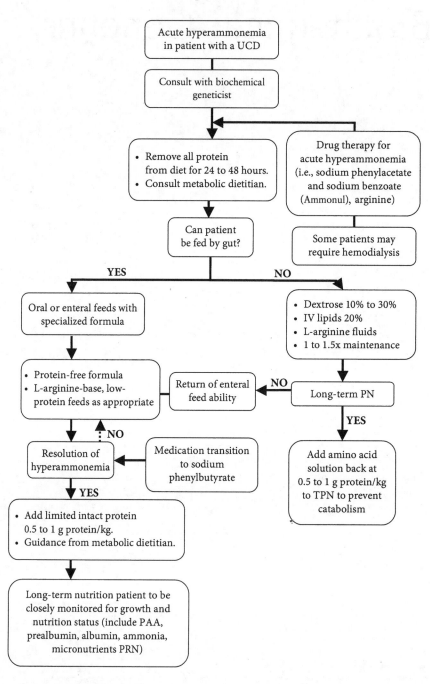

5.1 Urea Cycle Defects
Kelly McKean, Melissa Edwards

5.1.1 Name of Disorder

Urea cycle defects (UCD).

5.1.2 Clinical Definition

The urea cycle is the enzyme cycle whereby ammonia is converted to urea. Disorders of the urea cycle result from genetic defects in any one of the six enzymes that function in urea production (see nearby table).

5.1.3 How It Is Diagnosed

Increased plasma ammonia. In addition, plasma amino acids and urine organic acids and orotic acid, blood glucose, ketones, anion gap, and pH and CO_2 may be abnormal. Increased plasma citrulline, argininosuccinic acid, and arginine occur in citrullinemia, argininosuccinic acidemia, and argininemia, respectively.

5.1.4 Nutritional Implications

In acute hyperammonemia, protein intake elevates ammonia further. However, over-restriction of protein can result in body protein catabolism and can contribute to hyperammonemia.

Symbol	Prevalence/ Inheritance	Symptom Onset	Symptoms
N-acetylglutamate synthase deficiency (NAGS)	Rare Autosomal recessive	Symptoms occur shortly after birth. A partial deficiency may occur later in life following a stressful event such as an infection or a viral illness	Lethargy, vomiting, poor feeding, hyperventilation, enlarged liver, seizures
Carbamyl phosphate synthetase deficiency (CPS)	1:60,000 Autosomal recessive	Complete deficiency: 24–72 hours after birth Partial deficiency: Childhood	Lethargy, coma, seizures, vomiting, poor feeding, hyperventilation, hepatomegaly
Ornithine transcarbamylase deficiency (OTC)	1:30,000 X-linked	Hemizygote males: Onset in 24–72 hours after birth Heterozygote females: 10% are symptomatic in childhood	Lethargy, coma, seizures, vomiting, poor feeding, hyperventilation, hepatomegaly

Symbol	Prevalence/ Inheritance	Symptom Onset	Symptoms
Argininosuccinate synthetase deficiency (citrullinemia) (ASS)	1:60,000 Autosomal recessive	Complete deficiency: 24–72 hours after birth Partial deficiency: Childhood	Lethargy, coma, seizures, vomiting, poor feeding, hepatomegaly
Argininosuccinate lyase deficiency (argininosuccinic aciduria) (ASL)	1:70,000 Autosomal recessive	Complete deficiency: 24–72 hours after birth Partial deficiency: Childhood	Lethargy, seizures, vomiting, poor feeding, hyperventilation, hepatomegaly
Arginase deficiency (ARG)	Rare Autosomal recessive	Slower onset of symptoms than other UCDs Hyperammonemia is rare	Development delay, protein intolerance, spasticity, seizures, irritability, poor appetite and vomiting

National Urea Cycle Disorders Foundation Web site. Available at: http://www.nucdf.org/ucd.htm. Accessed April 30, 2011.

5.1.5   Pearls

- Lifelong nutrition therapy is focused on promoting protein anabolism during the chronic dietary restriction of protein as part of the treatment.
- High-quality protein is delivered through the use of medical metabolic formulas that contain essential amino acids (EAAs) to support amino acid/protein needs with reduced nitrogen load.
- The urea cycle not only makes urea but also arginine. Arginine becomes a conditionally EAA. Arginine is an important supplement for all urea cycle disorders except arginase deficiency. Citrulline may be used in OTC or CPS deficiency.
- Some common medical metabolic formulas are Cyclinex-1 (Abbott), Cyclinex-2 (Abbott), EAA supplement (Vitaflo), Essential Amino Acid Mix (Nutricia), WND-1 (Mead Johnson), and WND-2 (Mead Johnson).

Nutritional Algorithm for Maple Syrup Urine Disease (MSUD)

Maple Syrup Urine Disease (MSUD)

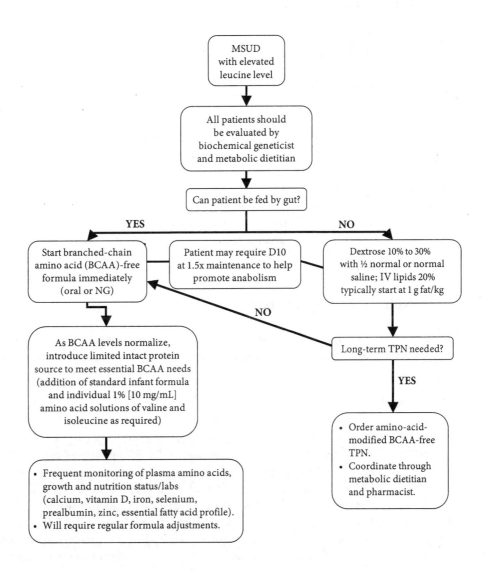

MSUD
with elevated
leucine level

All patients should
be evaluated by
biochemical geneticist
and metabolic dietitian

Can patient be fed by gut?

YES

NO

Start branched-chain
amino acid (BCAA)-free
formula immediately
(oral or NG)

Patient may require D10
at 1.5x maintenance to help
promote anabolism

Dextrose 10% to 30%
with ½ normal or normal
saline; IV lipids 20%
typically start at 1 g fat/kg

NO

As BCAA levels normalize,
introduce limited intact protein
source to meet essential BCAA needs
(addition of standard infant formula
and individual 1% [10 mg/mL]
amino acid solutions of valine and
isoleucine as required)

Long-term TPN needed?

YES

- Frequent monitoring of plasma amino acids,
  growth and nutrition status/labs
  (calcium, vitamin D, iron, selenium,
  prealbumin, zinc, essential fatty acid profile).
- Will require regular formula adjustments.

- Order amino-acid-
  modified BCAA-free
  TPN.
- Coordinate through
  metabolic dietitian
  and pharmacist.

5.2   Maple Syrup Urine Disease
Kelly McKean, Melissa Edwards

5.2.1   Name of Disorder

Maple syrup urine disease (MSUD).

5.2.2   Clinical Definition

Disorder of branched-chain amino acid (BCAA) metabolism; block in branched-chain α-ketoacid dehydrogenase complex.

5.2.3   How It Is Diagnosed

Abnormal plasma amino acids (elevated leucine, isoleucine, valine, alloisoleucine) and urine organic acids with abnormal branched-chain hydroxyacids and ketoacids.

5.2.4   Nutritional Implications

Lifelong restriction of leucine, isoleucine, and valine, likely requiring specialized low-protein foods. Supplemental medical formula that is free of BCAAs.

5.2.5   Pearls

- MSUD requires lifelong nutrition therapy.
- If MSUD patient is symptomatic (vomiting, lethargic), it is important to proceed immediately with IV hydration before obtaining laboratory results. Start an IV with D10 ½ normal saline run at 1.5 maintenance rate. If acidotic, give sodium bicarbonate per biochemical genetics team recommendations.
- If MSUD patient blood leucine is >800 μmol/L or if clinically indicated (excessive vomiting/neurologic compromise), pharmacy may need to order special total parenteral nutrition (free of branched-chain amino acids).

Nutritional Algorithm for Carbohydrate Metabolism Defects: Galactosemia

Galactosemia

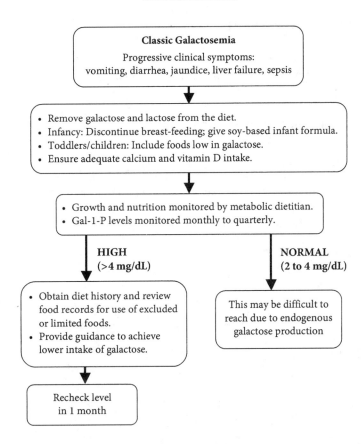

Classic Galactosemia

Progressive clinical symptoms:
vomiting, diarrhea, jaundice, liver failure, sepsis

- Remove galactose and lactose from the diet.
- Infancy: Discontinue breast-feeding; give soy-based infant formula.
- Toddlers/children: Include foods low in galactose.
- Ensure adequate calcium and vitamin D intake.

- Growth and nutrition monitored by metabolic dietitian.
- Gal-1-P levels monitored monthly to quarterly.

HIGH
(>4 mg/dL)

NORMAL
(2 to 4 mg/dL)

- Obtain diet history and review food records for use of excluded or limited foods.
- Provide guidance to achieve lower intake of galactose.

This may be difficult to reach due to endogenous galactose production

Recheck level in 1 month

5.3 Galactosemia

Kelly McKean, Melissa Edwards

5.3.1 Name of Disorder

Galactosemia.

5.3.2 Clinical Definition

Classic galactosemia is an inherited disorder of galactose metabolism that results from a defect in the enzyme galactose-1-phosphate uridyltransferase (GALT). The accumulation of galactose-1-phosphate (Gal-1-P) and galactose causes multiorgan disease (liver disease, cataracts, renal tubular dysfunction, growth failure, and ovarian dysfunction in females). Two other very rare forms of galactosemia exist that are due to deficiency in the enzymes galactokinase or uridine diphosphate-Gal-4-epimerase.

5.3.3   How It Is Diagnosed

Quantification of erythrocyte Gal-1-P and GALT activity. Classic galactosemia shows <1% GALT activity and markedly increased Gal-1-P.

5.3.4   Nutritional Implications

Early intervention with a galactose-restricted diet. No breast-feeding. Give powdered soy infant formula. The goal is to restrict galactose to the lowest amount compatible with a diet that is nutritionally adequate. Despite strict elimination of galactose from the diet, outcome is variable. Ensure adequate calcium and vitamin D intake.

Nutritional Algorithm for Carbohydrate Metabolism Defects: Glycogen Storage Disease (GSD) Types 1a and 1b

Glycogen Storage Disease (GSD) Types 1a and 1b

Glycogen Storage Disease Type 1a and 1b

Clinical symptoms: recurrent hypoglycemia, seizures, "doll face," hepatomegaly, bleeding abnormalities

- Limit sucrose, fructose, lactose and galactose.
- No breast milk. Provide ProSobee (soy) infant formula.
- Frequent feedings every 2 to 4 hours.
- Low-fat, high-complex-carbohydrate food choices.
- Ensure adequate calcium and vitamin D intake.
- Nocturnal feeding: intermittent PO feeds every 2 to 4 hours or continuous NG drip feeds.

- Raw cornstarch replaces some of the complex carbohydrates in the diet when pancreatic amylase enzyme is present (~12 months of age).
- Goal ranges from 1.25 to 2.5 g CHO/kg/feed based on blood glucose levels.

Growth and nutrition monitored by metabolic dietitian to include glucose, albumin, prealbumin, iron status, calcium, vitamin D, triglycerides, cholesterol, lactic acid and uric acid.

5.4 Glycogen Storage Disease Types 1a and 1b
Kelly McKean, Melissa Edwards

5.4.1 Name of Disorder

Glycogen storage disease (GSD) types 1a and 1b.

5.4.2 Clinical Definition

The GSDs are caused by deficiencies of enzymes that regulate the synthesis or degradation of glycogen. The enzyme defect between glucose-6-phosphate and glucose blocks both glycogenolysis and gluconeogenesis. GSD type 1a is due to a deficiency of the enzyme glucose-6-phosphatase, normally found in liver, kidney, and intestinal mucosa. GSD type 1b results from a defect in glucose-6-phosphate translocase, affecting transfer of glucose-6-phosphate into the endoplasmic reticulum. Hypoglycemia occurs when exogenous sources of glucose are exhausted.

5.4.3 How It Is Diagnosed

Liver biopsy and DNA analysis. Clinically suspected in individuals with hepatomegaly, growth retardation, bleeding tendency, severe neutropenia (type 1b), hypoglycemia, and increased lactate, uric acid, triglycerides, and transaminases.

5.4.4 Nutritional Implications

The goal is to prevent hypoglycemia and to normalize secondary metabolic abnormalities as possible. Two approaches (individually or in combination) are used: raw cornstarch therapy and nocturnal drip feedings of a carbohydrate-containing solution (drip feedings are started within 1 hour after last meal). Avoid prolonged fasting >5–7 hours. Some patients cannot tolerate fasting >3.5 hours. Limit food and medications containing sucrose, fructose, lactose, and galactose. No breast-feeding. ProSobee (Mead Johnson) formula is the only acceptable standard infant formula because it is lactose- and sucrose-free. Include low-fat complex carbohydrate food choices. Frequent feedings every 2–4 hours. Cornstarch is not recommended for use in infants <6 months old because pancreatic amylase activity has not reached normal adult activity; cornstarch therapy is typically started at 12 months of age.

Nutritional Algorithm for Carbohydrate Metabolism Defects: Hereditary Fructose Intolerance (HFI)

Hereditary Fructose Intolerance (HFI)

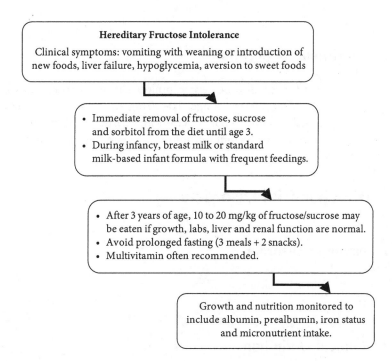

Hereditary Fructose Intolerance

Clinical symptoms: vomiting with weaning or introduction of new foods, liver failure, hypoglycemia, aversion to sweet foods

- Immediate removal of fructose, sucrose and sorbitol from the diet until age 3.
- During infancy, breast milk or standard milk-based infant formula with frequent feedings.

- After 3 years of age, 10 to 20 mg/kg of fructose/sucrose may be eaten if growth, labs, liver and renal function are normal.
- Avoid prolonged fasting (3 meals + 2 snacks).
- Multivitamin often recommended.

Growth and nutrition monitored to include albumin, prealbumin, iron status and micronutrient intake.

5.5   Hereditary Fructose Intolerance

Kelly McKean, Melissa Edwards

5.5.1   Name of Disorder

Hereditary fructose intolerance (HFI).

5.5.2   Clinical Definition

Deficiency in the activity of the enzyme fructose-1-phosphate aldolase (aldolase B); normally present in liver, intestine, and kidney cortex. Fructose-1-phosphate accumulates in tissues that contain fructokinase, which causes depletion of inorganic phosphate and adenosine-5′-triphosphate (ATP). Undiagnosed and untreated it will lead to liver and kidney impairment. Fructose-induced hypoglycemia results from inhibition of both gluconeogenesis and glycogenolysis.

5.5.3   How It Is Diagnosed

Molecular analysis of DNA or an enzyme assay of aldolase B activity in liver tissue obtained by liver biopsy.

5.5.4   Nutritional Implications

Diet free of all foods containing fructose, sucrose, and sorbitol until 3 years of age. After 3 years of age, 10–20 mg/kg of these sugars may be eaten if growth, labs, liver, and renal function are normal. Use breast milk or standard milk-based infant formula in infancy. Check the ingredients on modified formulas.

5.6   Mitochondrial Disorders

Kelly McKean, Melissa Edwards

5.6.1   Name of Disorder

Mitochondrial disorders.

5.6.2   Clinical Definition

A group of degenerative disorders characterized by impaired energy production by the mitochondria due to genetically based oxidative phosphorylation dysfunction. Organs typically affected are those with a high energy demand, including skeletal and cardiac muscle, endocrine organs, kidney, liver, nonmucosal components of the intestinal tract, retina, and the central nervous system. However, virtually any organ or tissue can be involved.

5.6.3   How It Is Diagnosed

Diagnosis is difficult due to the variable and often nonspecific presentation of these disorders, as well as from the absence of a reliable specific biomarker. Criteria are based on presence of muscular disease, central nervous system (CNS) disease, and multisystem involvement in addition to elevations of lactate, pyruvate in blood, urine or cerebrospinal fluid (CSF) and Kreb cycle intermediates in urine organic acid analysis. Often patients have abnormalities on magnetic resonance imaging (MRI) and MR spectroscopy. Muscle biopsy for histochemistry and electron microscopy with respiratory chain complex enzyme analysis is often helpful (however, a normal result does not preclude mitochondrial dysfunction).

5.6.4 Nutritional Implications

Vitamin "cocktail" treatment to boost cell function often includes coenzyme Q10, vitamin C, vitamin E, riboflavin, thiamin, niacin, creatine, lipoic acid, and L-carnitine. The goal of nutritional cofactor therapy is to increase mitochondrial ATP production and to slow the progression of clinical symptoms by protecting from cellular damage with antioxidants. There is widespread disparity regarding the effectiveness of the "cocktail" treatment. Avoid fasting. Small frequent meals may be better tolerated. Many patients may have already self-adjusted their diets based on foods they best tolerate. A complex carbohydrate snack before bedtime may be helpful. A diet high in fat and lower in carbohydrate is preferable in complex I deficiency and often trialed in patients with an unspecified mitochondrial disorder to see if there is subjective improvement.

5.6.5 Pearls

- Although individual vitamins and combinations of cofactors have been used widely in the treatment of patients with mitochondrial disorders, evidence of a significant effect on the course of the disease has not been demonstrated.
- Due to the diverse nature of these conditions, the evaluation of any nutritional therapy remains a challenge.
- Mitochondrial disease is underdiagnosed. Referral to a biochemical geneticist should always be made when signs and symptoms strongly suggest mitochondrial disease.

Nutritional Algorithm for Mitochondrial Disorder: Fatty Acid Oxidation Disorders (FAOD)

Fatty Acid Oxidation Disorder

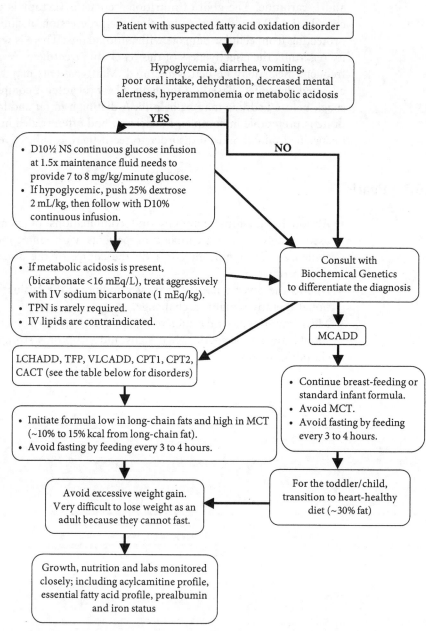

Patient with suspected fatty acid oxidation disorder

Hypoglycemia, diarrhea, vomiting, poor oral intake, dehydration, decreased mental alertness, hyperammonemia or metabolic acidosis

YES

NO

- D10½ NS continuous glucose infusion at 1.5x maintenance fluid needs to provide 7 to 8 mg/kg/minute glucose.
- If hypoglycemic, push 25% dextrose 2 mL/kg, then follow with D10% continuous infusion.

- If metabolic acidosis is present, (bicarbonate <16 mEq/L), treat aggressively with IV sodium bicarbonate (1 mEq/kg).
- TPN is rarely required.
- IV lipids are contraindicated.

Consult with Biochemical Genetics to differentiate the diagnosis

MCADD

LCHADD, TFP, VLCADD, CPT1, CPT2, CACT (see the table below for disorders)

- Continue breast-feeding or standard infant formula.
- Avoid MCT.
- Avoid fasting by feeding every 3 to 4 hours.

- Initiate formula low in long-chain fats and high in MCT (~10% to 15% kcal from long-chain fat).
- Avoid fasting by feeding every 3 to 4 hours.

For the toddler/child, transition to heart-healthy diet (~30% fat)

Avoid excessive weight gain. Very difficult to lose weight as an adult because they cannot fast.

Growth, nutrition and labs monitored closely; including acylcamitine profile, essential fatty acid profile, prealbumin and iron status

5.7 Fatty Acid Oxidation Disorders

Kelly McKean, Melissa Edwards

5.7.1 Name of Disorder

Fatty acid oxidation disorders (FAODs).

5.7.2 Clinical Definition

Fatty acids and potentially toxic derivatives accumulate because of a deficiency in one of the mitochondrial fatty acid oxidation enzymes. Fatty acid oxidation occurs during prolonged fasting and/or periods of increased energy demands (fever, stress) when energy production relies increasingly on fat metabolism.

5.7.3 How It Is Diagnosed

Elevated plasma acylcarnitines (see the nearby table) and the presence of urine organic acids. Diagnosis is confirmed by mutation analysis for the specific genes involved or by enzyme assay in cultured fibroblasts from a skin biopsy.

5.7.4 Nutritional Implications

- A low-fat, high-carbohydrate diet is recommended (see the table for modifications based on the enzyme defect).
- Plasma essential fatty acid levels are monitored to prevent deficiency.
- Avoid fasting in all disorders, with regular feedings during the day and limited overnight fasting. Raw cornstarch may be used before bedtime (1–1.5 g/kg) to prevent overnight hypoglycemia in infants >9–12 months of age (cornstarch is a complex carbohydrate that provides a slowly released source of glucose).
- In long chain fatty acid (LCFA) oxidation disorders the diet is supplemented with medium chain triglycerides (MCT) to provide an alternate energy source downstream of the enzymatic block and decrease LCFA oxidation. MCT is contraindicated in MCADD.

Fatty Acid Oxidation Disorder	Enzyme Missing or Inactive	Plasma Acylcarnitine Analysis	Nutrition Intervention
Medium-chain acyl-CoA dehydrogenase deficiency (MCADD)	Medium-chain acyl-CoA dehydrogenase	↑ C8 with lesser elevations in C6, C10	Avoid fasting, avoid MCT, and eat a moderately low-fat, heart-healthy diet (~30% fat)

Fatty Acid Oxidation Disorder	Enzyme Missing or Inactive	Plasma Acylcarnitine Analysis	Nutrition Intervention
Long-chain 3-hydroxy-acyl-CoA dehydrogenase deficiency (LCHADD)/ trifunctional protein deficiency (TFP)	Long-chain 3-hydroxy-acyl-CoA dehydrogenase/ trifunctional protein	↑ C16-OH ± ↑ C18:1-OH and other long-chain acylcarnitines	
Very-long-chain acyl-CoA dehydrogenase deficiency (VLCADD)	Very-long-chain acyl-CoA dehydrogenase	↑ C14:1 ± ↑ in other long-chain acylcarnitines	Avoid fasting, low long-chain fatty acids (~10–15% fat), and supplement with MCT
Carnitine palmitoyl transferase 1 deficiency (CPT 1)	Carnitine palmitoyl transferase 1	↑ C0 (free carnitine) with low or normal long-chain acylcarnitines	
Carnitine palmitoyl transferase 2 deficiency (CPT 2)/ carnitine acylcarnitine translocase deficiency (CACT)	Carnitine palmitoyl transferase 2/ carnitine acylcarnitine translocase	↑ C16 and/or C18:1	

5.7.5   Pearls

- Treatment includes avoiding fasting and catabolism, suppressing lipolysis, and providing carnitine supplementation. Carnitine may be low because fatty acids conjugate with carnitine and are excreted as acylcarnitine.
- Nutrition therapy is lifelong to support growth, development, and nutrition status and to prevent the accumulation of abnormal biochemical metabolites.
- Formulas high in MCT and low in long-chain fat, used for individuals with long-chain fatty acid disorders, include Lipistart (Vitaflo), Monogen (Nutricia), and Portagen (Mead Johnson).
- Use of oils with essential fatty acids may be needed if the formula and/or diet content is not adequate.
- Parents of children with diagnosed metabolic disorders know the early signs of decompensation in *their* children. Listen to them! Treat emergently.

Nutritional Algorithm for Organic Acidemia

Organic Acidemia

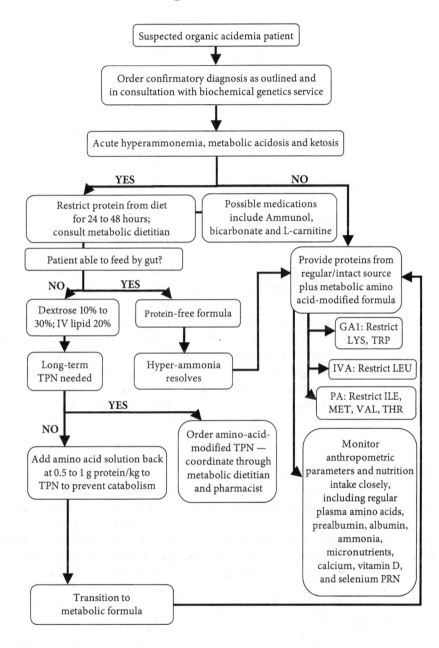

5.8   Organic Acidemia
Kelly McKean, Melissa Edwards

5.8.1   Name of Disorder

Organic acidemias (organic aciduria).

5.8.2   Clinical Definition

A group of metabolic disorders that disrupt normal amino acid metabolism.

5.8.3   How It Is Diagnosed

- **Glutaric acidemia (GA-1):** Plasma acylcarnitine with elevated C5-DC, elevated urinary glutaric acid, and 3-hydroxyglutaric acid. If these blood and urine studies are not diagnostic, further tests may be required (urinary glutaryl carnitine, with elevated 3-hydroxyglutaric acid, enzyme assay in fibroblasts, and genetic molecular analysis).
- **Isovaleric acidemia (IVA):** Plasma acylcarnitine with elevated C5, increased urinary isovalerylglycine. Urine acyl glycine and acylcarnitine analysis may also be informative. Diagnose with DNA sequencing. Mild forms exist.
- **Methylmalonic acidemia (MMA) and propionic acidemia (PA):** Plasma acylcarnitine with increased C3, increased plasma glycine, and increased urinary metabolites (3-hydroxyproprionic acid, methylcitric acid) characteristic of propionic acidemia or methylmalonic acidemia. Plasma total homocysteine is elevated in the cobalamin C, D, and F deficiencies.

5.8.4   Nutritional Implications

In acute decompensation, patient will likely be acidotic and have hyperammonemia. Protein intake will elevate ammonia further while overrestriction of protein can result in body protein catabolism and can contribute to hyperammonemia. Gradual reintroduction of intact (regular infant formula or breast milk) and medically modified protein will be required to meet nutritional needs.

5.8.5   Pearls

- Lifelong nutrition therapy is focused on promoting protein anabolism during the chronic dietary restriction of protein as part of the treatment.
- High-quality protein is delivered through the use of medical metabolic formulas that contain amino acids that are able to be metabolized, with restriction of "offending amino acids" depending on patient's disorder.

- Some common medical metabolic formulas:
  - GA-1 are Glutarex-1 (Abbott), Glutarex-2 (Abbott), GA (Mead Johnson), and X Lys X Trp (Nutricia).
  - IVA are I-Valex-1 (Abbott), I-Valex-2 (Abbott), LMD (Mead Johnson), and X Leu (Nutricia).
  - MMA/PA are Propimex-1 (Abbott), Propimex-2 (Abbott), OA1 (Mead Johnson), and OA2 (Mead Johnson).
- Many times patients with these disorders require protein-free nutrition modulars to meet calories and nutrient needs, such as PFD-1 and PFD-2 (Mead Johnson).

5.8.6   Clinical Considerations

- A GA-1 neonate is usually macrocephalic but otherwise asymptomatic. Later signs include possible sudden onset of dystonia and athetosis due to irreversible striatal damage, metabolic ketoacidosis, and failure to thrive.
- IVA presents in the neonate with metabolic ketoacidosis, a "sweaty feet" odor, dehydration, hyperammonemia, ketonuria, vomiting, hypoglycemia, and failure to thrive. Milder variants without neonatal illness exist. Long-term prognosis of IVA is good with appropriate therapy.
- PA and severe cases of MMA typically present in the neonate with metabolic ketoacidosis, dehydration, hyperammonemia, ketonuria, vomiting, hypoglycemia, and failure to thrive. Long-term complications are common; early treatment is likely lifesaving. Cobalamin disorders types C, D, and F typically do not have significant metabolic acidosis.

References

Acosta PB. *Nutrition Management of Patients with Inherited Metabolic Disorders.* Sudbury, MA: Jones and Bartlett; 2010.

Acosta PB, Yannicelli S. *Ross Metabolic Formula System Nutrition Support Protocols,* 4th ed. Columbus, OH: Ross Products Division, Abbott Laboratories; 2001.

Acosta PB, Yannicelli S, Ryan AS, et al. Nutritional therapy improves growth and protein status of children with a urea cycle enzyme defect. *Mol Genet Metab.* 2005;86(4):448–455.

Morton DH, Strauss KA, Robinson DL, Puffenberger EG, Kelley RI. Diagnosis and treatment of maple syrup disease: a study of 36 patients. *Pediatrics.* 2002; 109(6):999–1008.

Newborn screening ACT Sheets and Confirmatory Algorithms. Available at: http://www.acmg.net/resources/policies/ACT/condition-analyte-links.htm. Accessed June 2010.

New England Consortium of Metabolic Programs Acute Illness Protocols: Fatty Acid Oxidation Disorders. Available at: http://newenglandconsortium.org/for-professionals/acute-illness-protocols/fatty-acid-oxidation-disorders. Accessed June 2010.

Singh RH. Nutrition management of patient with urea cycle disorders. *J Inherit Metab Dis.* 2007;30(6):880–887.

Singh RH. *Nutritional Management of Urea Cycle Disorders: A Practical Reference for Clinicians*. Atlanta, GA: Emory University Press; 2006.

Spiekerkoetter U, Lindner M, Santer R, et al. Treatment recommendations in long-chain fatty acid oxidation defects: consensus from a workshop. *J Inherit Metab Dis*. 2009;32(4):498–505.

Strauss KA, Wardley B, Robinson D, et al. Classical maple syrup urine disease and brain development: principles of management and formula design. *Mol Genet Metab*. 2010;99(4):333–345.

Chapter 6
Nephrology

6.1 Nephrotic Syndrome
Peggy Solan, Kirsten Thompson

6.1.1 Name of Disorder

Nephrotic syndrome.

6.1.2 Clinical Definition

Nephrotic syndrome is not a disease but a constellation of clinical findings common to a number of renal disorders: proteinuria >50 mg/kg per 24 hours (>40 mg/m^2 per hour or a protein-to-creatinine ratio >2); hypoalbuminemia (serum albumin <3 g/dL); edema and hypercholesterolemia are commonly present.

6.1.3 How It Is Diagnosed

Test for serum albumin, creatinine, blood urea nitrogen (BUN), electrolytes, and urinalysis. A kidney biopsy may be performed. Other labs of interest include a thyroid panel, complete blood count (CBC), calcium, 25-OH vitamin D, and a fasting lipid panel.

6.1.4 Nutritional Implications

Low sodium (Na+) diet. At risk for hyperglycemia and hyperlipidemia.

Pediatric Nutrition Handbook: An Algorithmic Approach, First Edition. Edited by David L. Suskind and Polly Lenssen.
© 2011 Blackwell Publishing Ltd. Published 2011 by Blackwell Publishing Ltd.

6.1.5   General Nutrition Guidelines

1. **Low-sodium diet:**
   - 1–3 mEq/kg, or 23–69 mg/kg.
   - The level of restriction depends on severity of edema and/or presence of hypertension.
2. **If patient is edematous,** consider fluid restriction.
3. **Ensure adequate calcium and vitamin D intake;** supplement as indicated.
4. **If patient is on a prednisone treatment,** consider additional calcium and vitamin D. If hyperglycemia is present, consider a carbohydrate-controlled diet as needed.
5. **If hyperlipidemia is present,** recommend a low-fat diet as appropriate and if able to meet caloric needs.

6.1.6   Pearls

- A high-protein diet is generally not recommended because it causes increased urinary protein losses.
- The edema associated with nephrotic syndrome can be so severe as to limit mobility.
- The reason for the increased hepatic production of lipoproteins during the nephrotic state is not entirely understood, but it may be linked to low plasma oncotic pressure or defects in lipoprotein catabolism.

Nutritional Algorithm for Chronic Kidney Disease (CKD)

Chronic Kidney Disease (CKD)

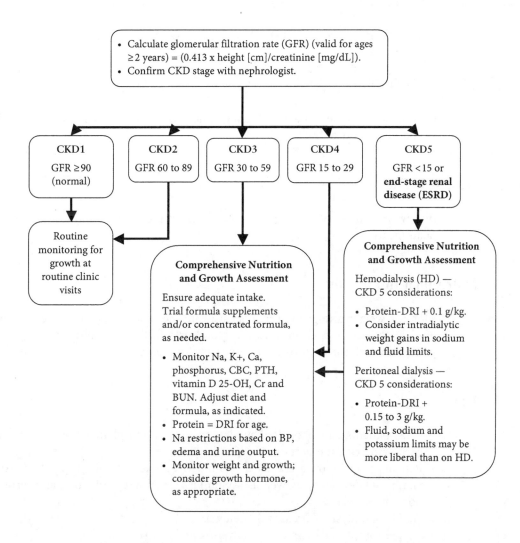

- Calculate glomerular filtration rate (GFR) (valid for ages ≥2 years) = (0.413 x height [cm]/creatinine [mg/dL]).
- Confirm CKD stage with nephrologist.

CKD1

GFR ≥90 (normal)

CKD2

GFR 60 to 89

CKD3

GFR 30 to 59

CKD4

GFR 15 to 29

CKD5

GFR <15 or **end-stage renal disease (ESRD)**

Routine monitoring for growth at routine clinic visits

Comprehensive Nutrition and Growth Assessment

Ensure adequate intake. Trial formula supplements and/or concentrated formula, as needed.

- Monitor Na, K+, Ca, phosphorus, CBC, PTH, vitamin D 25-OH, Cr and BUN. Adjust diet and formula, as indicated.
- Protein = DRI for age.
- Na restrictions based on BP, edema and urine output.
- Monitor weight and growth; consider growth hormone, as appropriate.

Comprehensive Nutrition and Growth Assessment

Hemodialysis (HD) — CKD 5 considerations:

- Protein-DRI + 0.1 g/kg.
- Consider intradialytic weight gains in sodium and fluid limits.

Peritoneal dialysis — CKD 5 considerations:

- Protein-DRI + 0.15 to 3 g/kg.
- Fluid, sodium and potassium limits may be more liberal than on HD.

6.2   Chronic Kidney Disease
Peggy Solan, Kirsten Thompson

6.2.1   Name of Disorder

Chronic kidney disease (CKD).

6.2.2   Clinical Definition

Chronic irreversible changes in kidney structure/function, usually with reduced glomerular filtration rate.

6.2.3   How It Is Diagnosed

Biopsy, creatinine, BUN, electrolyte panel, renal ultrasound, and urine protein quantification.

6.2.4   Nutritional Implications

Monitor weight and growth trends. Institute the following diet restrictions as needed: sodium restriction based on blood pressure, edema and urine output, potassium and phosphorus restriction based on labs.

6.2.5   Pearls

- Most patients take phosphate binders to control phosphate levels (sevelamer carbonate, calcium acetate, $CaCO_3$).
- Patients may be on a standard vitamin D supplement due to 25 hydroxy vitamin D deficiency as well as a vitamin D analog to regulate parathyroid hormone levels.
  - a. Hemodialysis: Paricalcitol (Zemplar)
  - b. Peritoneal dialysis and predialysis: Calcitriol (Rocaltrol)
- Dialysis patients need a water-soluble vitamin with extra folate (Nephro-Vite, Nephronex) to replace vitamins lost with dialysis. Avoid supplements with vitamin A.

Nutritional Algorithm for Kidney Transplant

Kidney Transplant

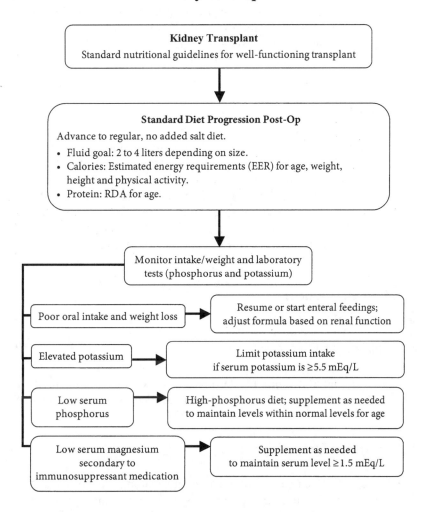

Kidney Transplant
Standard nutritional guidelines for well-functioning transplant

Standard Diet Progression Post-Op
Advance to regular, no added salt diet.
- Fluid goal: 2 to 4 liters depending on size.
- Calories: Estimated energy requirements (EER) for age, weight, height and physical activity.
- Protein: RDA for age.

Monitor intake/weight and laboratory tests (phosphorus and potassium)

Poor oral intake and weight loss → Resume or start enteral feedings; adjust formula based on renal function

Elevated potassium → Limit potassium intake if serum potassium is ≥5.5 mEq/L

Low serum phosphorus → High-phosphorus diet; supplement as needed to maintain levels within normal levels for age

Low serum magnesium secondary to immunosuppressant medication → Supplement as needed to maintain serum level ≥1.5 mEq/L

6.3 Kidney Transplant

Peggy Solan, Kirsten Thompson

6.3.1 Name of Disorder

Kidney transplant, early posttransplant phase.

6.3.2 Clinical Definition

The transplant of a kidney into a patient with end-stage renal disease, usually classified as deceased donor or living donor transplant, depending on organ source.

6.3.3   Nutritional Implications

Recommend a high-fluid, no-added-salt (3 g Na/day) regular diet. Possibly restrict potassium because of drug–nutrient interactions. Encourage foods high in magnesium due to magnesium wasting related to medications. Patients may experience phosphate wasting and a high phosphorus diet with supplementation is commonly needed.

6.3.4   Pearls

- Optimize calcium and vitamin D intake; supplement as needed. Ongoing concerns for renal osteodystrophy posttransplant. Continue to monitor vitamin D and parathyroid hormone levels as outpatient.
- Limit intake of refined sugars if hyperglycemic.
- Restrict sodium to 2 mEq/kg per day or a maximum of 2 g/day if hypertension or edema is present.
- Refer to the CKD section for poorly functioning transplant.

6.4   Hypertension

Peggy Solan, Kirsten Thompson

6.4.1   Name of Disorder

Blood pressure is >95th percentile for age, gender, and height on three different occasions. Prehypertension is defined as blood pressure >90th percentile.

6.4.2   Clinical Definition

Comparison of blood pressure readings to normal ranges; recommendations for 24-hour ambulatory blood pressure measurements. Other tests may include BUN, creatinine, electrolytes, CBC, fasting glucose and lipid levels, urinalysis, renal ultrasound, and echocardiogram.

6.4.3   Nutritional Implications

Recommend a low-sodium diet, evaluate body mass index (BMI), and initiate guidelines for weight management as indicated.

If blood pressure >90th percentile:

- Recommend a low-sodium diet, <2000 mg/day.
- Counsel regarding caffeine, energy drinks, and herbal supplements that may elevate blood pressure.
- Review DASH (Dietary Approaches to Stop Hypertension) diet.

If BMI >85th percentile:

- Implement American Academy of Pediatrics guidelines for overweight/obesity (see Chapter 8 on obesity).

6.4.4   Pearls

- The DASH diet has been shown to reduce blood pressure in adolescents. Recommendations include increasing fruits and vegetables, increasing fiber, using low-fat dairy products and limiting total fat intake. See www.nhlbi.nih.gov/health/public/heart/hbp/dash/dash_brief.pdf.
- Lifestyle modifications for hypertension management should also include activity goals.

Chapter 7

Neurology

7.1 Antiepileptic Drug–Nutrient Interactions

Elaine Cumbie, Marta Mazzanti

Drug Mechanism of Action	Drug–Nutrient Interactions	Nutrition Intervention	Routine Lab Monitoring
ACTH: corticosteroids	1. Interferes with vitamin D and folate metabolism 2. Increased risk for bone demineralization due to low serum vitamin D values, decreased uptake of calcium from the gut, and increased osteoclast activity 3. Increased appetite with rapid weight gain 4. Impaired glucose tolerance 5. Foods high in sodium are preferred/eaten, resulting in increased fluid retention and weight gain 6. Muscle wasting; reduction of protein stores	1. Monitor appetite and weight gain 2. Monitor blood glucose 3. Monitor growth and potential for linear growth 4. Consider multivitamin (MVI) 5. Adequate hydration is important; may need fluids 6. Sodium retention: May need sodium, potassium, protein, calcium, phosphorus, zinc, vitamins A/B_6/C/D, folate 7. Avoid high-dose vitamin C or E 8. Prescreen for vitamin D deficiency; if low or low normal, give 1000 IU daily of OTC vitamin D; rescreen in 3 months	1. Complete blood count (CBC) with differential 2. Liver enzymes with long-term use 3. Albumin and prealbumin 4. Calcium, electrolytes 5. Serum glucose 6. Vitamin D

Pediatric Nutrition Handbook: An Algorithmic Approach, First Edition. Edited by David L. Suskind and Polly Lenssen.
© 2011 Blackwell Publishing Ltd. Published 2011 by Blackwell Publishing Ltd.

Drug Mechanism of Action	Drug–Nutrient Interactions	Nutrition Intervention	Routine Lab Monitoring
Phenytoin (Dilantin): Na+ channel modulation	1. Interferes with metabolism of vitamins D, K, B$_{12}$, and folate 2. Folate required for drug metabolism 3. Low albumin can increase risk of drug toxicity 4. Gingival hyperplasia may affect chewing and tolerance of foods and cause weight loss 5. Inhibits metabolism of vitamin K; consider supplement	1. Monitor hydration 2. Monitor weight 3. Consider MVI; folate, vitamin K, and vitamin D supplementation recommended when drug is initiated 4. Prescreen for vitamin D deficiency; if low or low normal, give 1000 IU daily of OTC vitamin D; rescreen in 3 months 5. Hold tube feeding 1–2 hours pre- and postfeed 6. Separate calcium and magnesium supplements by 2 hours 7. No medications with alcohol or caffeine 8. Take with food 9. Avoid high-dose vitamins B$_6$, C, and E 10. Encourage good dental hygiene	1. CBC with differential 2. Vitamin D, baseline and follow-up at 3 months 3. Liver enzymes 4. Follow albumin as phenytoin is highly protein-bound; low albumin can lead to drug toxicity: If low, check free drug levels 5. Serum or urine homocystine levels are important; homocystinuria and/or homocystinemia is diagnostic for folate deficiency
Carbamazepine (Tegretol): Na+ channel modulation	1. Possible weight gain: May decrease compliance in teens 2. Nausea 3. Increase risk of dental caries 4. Accelerates the metabolism of folate and biotin, possibly causing deficiency 5. Interferes with metabolism of vitamin D	1. Monitor hydration, weight, and nutritional status 2. Consider MVI (biotin, folate) 3. Avoid high-dose vitamin C or E supplementation 4. Take with food 5. No medications with alcohol or caffeine 6. Encourage good dental hygiene 7. Prescreen for vitamin D deficiency; if low or low normal, give 1000 IU daily of OTC vitamin D; rescreen in 3 months	1. CBC with differential, baseline and periodically 2. Electrolytes and blood urea nitrogen (BUN) 3. Liver enzymes and lipids 4. Serum or urine homocystine levels are important; homocystinuria and/or homocystinemia concerning for folate deficiency 5. Vitamin D
Oxcarbazepine (Trileptal): Na+ channel modulation	1. May cause nausea, vomiting, appetite alteration, and weight change 2. May aggravate gastroesophageal reflux disease 3. Possible blood glucose 4. Accelerates the metabolism of folate and biotin 5. Interferes with metabolism of vitamin D	1. Monitor hydration; may need to increase fluids and fiber 2. Consider MVI (biotin, folate) 3. Monitor weight 4. Blood glucose 5. No medications with alcohol or caffeine 6. Prescreen for vitamin D deficiency; if low or low normal, give 1000 IU daily of vitamin D; rescreen in 3 months	1. Electrolytes 2. Liver enzymes 3. CBC with differential 4. Serum or urine are homocystine levels important; homocystinuria and/or homocystinemia are concerning for folate deficiency 5. Vitamin D

Drug Mechanism of Action	Drug–Nutrient Interactions	Nutrition Intervention	Routine Lab Monitoring
Lamotrigine (Lamictal): Na+/Ca+ channel modulation	1. May cause nausea, vomiting, appetite alteration 2. May interfere with folate metabolism in long-term use 3. Interferes with metabolism of vitamin D	1. Monitor hydration; may need increased fluids 2. Monitor weight 3. Consider MVIs 4. Consider folate supplement with long-term use 5. Prescreen for vitamin D deficiency; if low or low normal, give 1000 IU daily of vitamin D; rescreen in 3 months	1. CBC with differential 2. Serum or urine homocystine levels are important; homocystinuria and/or homocystinemia is concerning for folate deficiency 3. Vitamin D
Zonisamide (Zonegran): carbonic anhydrase inhibitor	1. Can cause kidney stones 2. Can cause anorexia 3. Can cause metabolic acidosis and anhydrosis with dehydration 4. Can cause aplastic anemia 5. Interferes with metabolism of vitamin D	1. Monitor hydration, increase fluids to prevent renal stones, increase fiber 2. Monitor weight 3. Take with food 4. Avoid high-dose vitamin C or E 5. Prescreen for vitamin D deficiency; if low or low normal, give 1000 IU daily of OTC vitamin D; rescreen in 3 months	1. Electrolytes with BUN, creatinine 2. Alkaline phosphatase and liver enzymes 3. CBC
Valproic acid (Depacon, Depakene, Depakote): GABA system; Na+/Ca+ channel modulation	1. Appetite alteration; weight change 2. Increase blood glucose 3. Highly protein-bound; low albumin can increase risk of drug toxicity 4. Carnitine facilitates metabolism, increased use may lead to possible carnitine deficiency 5. Selenium, zinc, copper deficiency	1. Monitor hydration and weight 2. Take with food 3. Avoid high-dose vitamin C or E 4. Consider carnitine supplement for long-term use 5. Consider MVI 6. Selenium, supplement if low blood levels 7. Prescreen for vitamin D deficiency; if low or low normal, give 1000 IU daily of OTC vitamin D; rescreen in 3 months	1. Electrolytes 2. Liver enzymes with alkaline phosphatase 3. CBC with differential 4. Albumin: if low, check free drug level 5. Carnitine profile 6. Selenium, zinc, copper levels 7. Serum or urine homocystine levels are important; homocystinuria and/or homocystinemia is concerning for folate deficiency 8. Vitamin D
Felbamate (Felbatol) (rarely used): Glutamate receptors; GABA system; Na+/Ca+ channel modulation	1. Aplastic anemia 2. Weight loss	1. Monitor weight 2. Consider MVI 3. Monitor hydration; may need to increase fluids and fiber 4. Glucose 5. Prescreen for vitamin D deficiency; if low or low normal, give 1000 IU daily of vitamin D; rescreen in 3 months	1. CBC with differential 2. Electrolytes 3. Liver enzymes including alkaline phosphatase 4. Serum glucose

Drug Mechanism of Action	Drug–Nutrient Interactions	Nutrition Intervention	Routine Lab Monitoring
Topiramate (Topamax): Glutamate receptors; GABA system; Na+/Ca+ channel modulation	1. Appetite alteration 2. Weight loss 3. Nausea and vomiting 4. Kidney stones 5. Metabolic acidosis, anhydrosis with dehydration	1. Monitor hydration and weight 2. Monitor intake 3. Limit caffeine 4. Encourage increased fluids 5. Prescreen for vitamin D deficiency; if low or low normal, give 1000 IU daily of OTC vitamin D; rescreen in 3 months	1. Liver enzymes 2. Creatinine and BUN (renal function) 3. Electrolytes 4. CBC with differential 5. Vitamin D
Ethosuximide (Zarontin) : Na+/Ca+ channel modulation	1. Appetite alteration 2. Weight loss 3. Increased risk of dental caries 4. Possible interference with metabolism of folate	1. Monitor intake and weight 2. Consider MVI 3. May need to increase fluids and fiber 4. Take with food 5. Extra folate may be needed 6. Prescreen for vitamin D deficiency; if low or low normal, give 1000 IU daily of vitamin D; rescreen in 3 months	1. Liver enzymes 2. CBC with differential 3. BUN/creatinine 4. Vitamin D
Gabapentin (Neurontin): Ca+ channel modulation; GABA system	1. Appetite alteration 2. Weight loss 3. Increased risk of dental caries	1. Monitor intake, weight and hydration 2. Separate calcium and magnesium supplements by >2 hours 3. Prescreen for vitamin D deficiency; if low or low normal, give 1000 IU daily of vitamin D; rescreen in 3 months 4. Calcium and magnesium may bind to drug, decreasing absorption	1. Vitamin D
Levetiracetam (Keppra): neurotransmitter release modulation; Ca+ channel modulation; GABA system	1. Appetite alteration 2. Weight loss 3. Increased risk of dental caries	1. Monitor intake, weight and hydration 2. May need increased fluids and fiber 3. Consider MVI 4. Take with food	1. CBC with differential

Drug Mechanism of Action	Drug–Nutrient Interactions	Nutrition Intervention	Routine Lab Monitoring
Phenobarbital: Ca+ channel modulation; GABA system; glutamate receptors	1. Aplastic anemia 2. Osteomalacia with long-term use 3. Decreased drug effect with high doses of vitamin B_6 4. Delayed gastric emptying 5. Megaloblastic anemia 6. Decreased absorption of vitamins B_{12}, folate and D, as well as calcium	1. Monitor intake, weight, and hydration 2. Avoid >80 mg vitamin B_6 3. Assure adequate vitamins B_6, B_{12}, C, D, folate, and calcium; may need supplementation 4. MVI	1. CBC with differential 2. Liver enzymes and renal function; folate 3. Vitamin B_{12} 4. Bone mineral density if long-term use 5. Magnesium 6. Serum or urine homocystine levels are important; homocystinuria and/or homocystinemia is concerning for folate deficiency 7. Vitamin D
Primidone (Mysoline): Ca+ channel modulation; GABA system; glutamate receptors	1. Appetite decrease 2. Interferes with vitamin D and folate metabolism	1. Monitor intake and hydration 2. Consider MVI 3. May need increased fluids 4. Avoid high-dose vitamins C and E 5. Vitamin D as needed	1. CBC with differential 2. Liver enzymes 3. Serum or urine homocystine levels are important; homocystinuria and/or homocystinemia is concerning for folate deficiency 4. Folate 5. Vitamin D
Benzodiazepines (Clobazam, Clorazepate, Diazepam, Lorazepam, Midazolam, Nitrazepam): GABA-mediated mechanisms	1. Appetite decrease 2. Weight gain 3. Anemia	1. Monitor intake and hydration 2. May need increased fluids 3. Take with food 4. Avoid high-dose vitamins C and E	1. CBC with differential 2. Monitor hepatic and renal function
Vigabatrin (Sabril): GABA-mediated mechanisms	1. Weight increase 2. Diarrhea	1. Monitor intake	1. Electrolytes

References

Burke PK, Roche-Dudek M, Roche-Klemma K. *Drug-Nutrient Resource.* 5th ed. Riverside, IL: Roche Dietitians; 2003.

Nutritional Algorithm for Ketogenic Diet (KD) Therapy Plan

- Referral by epileptologist.
- Preadmission work-up with a minimum of 3 outpatient visits.
- Conversion of medication to lowest carbohydrate form.
- Development of low-carbohydrate meal plan for orally fed children and formula Rx for TF determining the formula prescription.
- Nutritional goals: 75% to 100% of estimated calorie needs, 100% to 110% of estimated fluid needs; 100% of estimated protein needs.

Traditional Method
- Constant ratio (e.g., 3:1) with increasing calories.
- Day 1: 1/3 of kcal goal.
- Day 2: 2/3 of kcal goal.
- Day 3: full kcal.

Modified Method
- Constant calories with increasing ratio (e.g., 3:1).
- Day 1: 2:1 ratio.
- Day 2: 2.5:1 ratio.
- Day 3: 3:1 ratio.

Monitoring daily labs include electrolytes, glucose and B-hydroxybutyrate

Blood sugar every 6 to 12 hours

Hydration Status
- In and outs.
- Weights.

Result	Intervention	Recheck Glucose
Glucose 30-40 mg/dL, patient alert and well (any age).	None	2 hours
Patient younger than 1 year		
If patient symptomatic, regardless blood glucose.	Give 7.5 mL Juice*.	1 hour
Glucose less than 30 mg/dL.	Give 7.5 mL Juice*.	1 hour
If Glucose less than prior measurement or symptomatic 1 hour after juice.	Give 7.5 mL Juice*. Call Neurology ARNP (day)/hospitalist (night).	1 hour
Patient seizing or unresponsive.	D10 10mL/kg IV STAT. Call Neurology ARNP (day)/hospitalist (night) STAT.	30 minutes
Patient older than 1 year		
If patient symptomatic, regardless blood glucose levels.	Give 15 mL Juice* (weight less than or equal to 20 kg). Give 30 mL Juice* (weight greater than 20 kg).	1 hour
Glucose less than 30mg/dL, patient symptomatic.	Give 15 mL Juice* (weight less than or equal to 20 kg). Give 30 mL Juice* (weight greater than 20 kg).	1 hour
If Glucose less than prior measurement or symptomatic 1 hour after juice.	Give 15 mL Juice* (weight less than or equal to 20 kg). Give 30 mL Juice* (weight greater than 20 kg). Call Neurology ARNP (day)/hospitalist (night).	1 hour
Patient seizing or unresponsive.	D10 10mL/kg IV STAT. Call Neurology ARNP (day)/hospitalist (night) STAT.	30 minutes

*Juice: Apple/orange juice given PO/GT.

If patient not meeting fluid needs, initiate ½ NS

Metabolic Acidosis
- Clinical signs/symptoms include nausea, vomiting, lethargy and refusal to eat.
- Labs will show low CO_2, increased anion gap and increased B-hydroxybutyrate.

- Administration of baking soda; mix with H_2O or formula (¼ to ½ tsp/day in 2 to 3 doses/day).
- Intravenous fluids with bicarbonate.
- Administration of 15 to 30 mL of orange juice or apple juice.
- Lowering of diet ratio.
- Adding calories.

Constipation → Treat with Miralax, Fleet enema or glycine suppository

Improved seizure controlled at 3 months

NO → Discontinue diet

YES → Continue diet for minimum of 2 years

Discharge with close follow-up monitoring

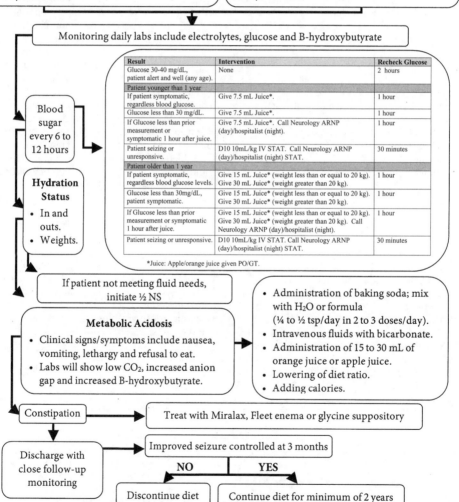

7.2 Ketogenic Diet Therapy Plan
Elaine Cumbie, Marta Mazzanti

7.2.1 Name of Treatment

The ketogenic diet (KD) is an established, effective, nonpharmacologic treatment for many types of epilepsy. It is most effective in controlling absence, atonic, myoclonic seizures, and infantile spasms in approximately a third of children who have been unable to control them with medications. The diet works by inducing and maintaining ketosis, simulating the metabolic effects of fasting. Ketones are thought to have an anticonvulsant action; however, the exact mechanism of the diet's anticonvulsant effects is not known. Ketones are the by-product of fat metabolism. The KD requires an experienced KD team, including a physician/advanced registered nurse practitioner, nurse, dietitian, and social worker.

7.2.2 Clinical Definition

Very low-carbohydrate diet with ratio of fat grams to combined grams of carbohydrate and protein (for example, 4:1 ratio = 4g fat for every 1g of protein and carbohydrate combined).

7.2.3 Nutritional Implications

Delayed growth, constipation, potential decreased bone mineral density, risk of kidney stones, increased triglycerides, potential vitamin D deficiency, nausea and vomiting.

7.2.4 Pearls

- Do not order or give carbohydrates in any medication or food.
- Do not give IV fluids with dextrose or lactated Ringer's. If patient is not meeting fluid needs, initiate ½ normal saline. Inadvertent dextrose administration can result in seizures.
- Consult the nutrition notes, pharmacy, and Safe List before ordering or administering medications or food.
- Diet intolerance is common during illness, resulting in metabolic acidosis and the need to modify the diet prescription. Provide a liquid diet in the form of ketogenic formula (KetoCal) and/or eggnog. If the diet is poorly tolerated, dilute to half to quarter of calories.
- For all medications order the lowest carbohydrate form available. Contact pharmacy or ketogenic RD for help.

References

Kinsman SL, Vining EP, Quaskey SA, Mellits D, Freeman JM. Efficacy of the ketogenic diet for intractable seizure disorders: review of 58 cases. *Epilepsia.* 1992;33(6): 1132–1136.

Phelps SJ, Collin A, Hovinga DF, Rose CV, Olsen-Creasy K. The ketogenic diet in pediatric epilepsy. *Nutr Clin Pract.* 1998;13(6):267–282.

Vining EP, Freeman JM, Ballaban-Gil K, et al. A multicenter study of the efficacy of the ketogenic diet. *Arch Neurol.* 1998;55(11):1433–1437.

Additional Resources

Internet

Charlie Foundation http://www.charliefoundation.org

Epilepsy Foundation of America http://www.efa.org

Book

Freeman J, Kossoff EH, Freeman JB, Kelly MT. *The Ketogenic Diet: A Treatment for Children and Others with Epilepsy.* New York, NY: Demos Medical Publishing; 2007.

Chapter 8

Obesity

Nutritional Algorithm for Obesity

Obesity

Calculate and Plot BMI Percentile for Age and Gender

1. Assess growth trajectory.
2. Update family medical history, patient's medical history and lab tests.
3. Assess sedentary time, physical activity and eating habits.
4. Assess patient and family concern and motivation.

All patients screened
for risk every year

Patient and Family Counseling

- Review any risks.
- Praise positive behaviors.
- Use motivational interviewing to elicit reasons to change.

Intervention

Patient advances through stages of treatment based
on age, risk factors and motivation of the family

Stage 1	Stage 2	Stage 3	Stage 4
Prevention plus: Target behaviors: • Eat breakfast daily. • Have family meals. • Encourage breast-feeding. • Do 60 minutes of physical activity each day. • Limit on-screen time (i.e., television or computer) to 2 hours or less per day. • Limit intake of sugar-sweetened beverages.	Structural weight management: Stage 1 plus support and structure provided to child/family individually or as a group; registered dietitian (RD) counseling	Comprehensive multidisciplinary team management: Weekly visits for 8 to 12 weeks and monthly visits thereafter to maintain habits; team may include medical provider, behavioral counselor, RD and exercise specialist	Tertiary care: Intervention may include medications, very low-calorie diet, or surgery; multidisciplinary team essential

8.1 Obesity

Heather Paves

8.1.1 Name of Disorder

Overweight and obesity.

8.1.2 Clinical Definition

Overweight is defined as between the 85th and 94th percentiles of body mass index (BMI) for age and gender; obesity is defined as >95th percentile BMI for age and gender on the Centers for Disease Control and Prevention (CDC) growth grids.

8.1.3 How It Is Diagnosed

Overweight and obesity are as just defined, but their diagnoses also need to take into account BMI trajectory over time, parental obesity, family medical history, current diet, and physical activity behaviors.

8.1.4 Nutritional Implications

More common comorbid conditions include sleep apnea, insulin resistance, type 2 diabetes, hyperlipidemia, hypertension, nonalcoholic steatohepatitis, depression, orthopedic conditions, and polycystic ovarian syndrome.

8.1.5 Pearls

- BMI is a screening tool for overweight and obesity. Integrate other clinical information such as growth trends and family history to determine associated medical risks for overweight or obesity.
- The clinical terms *overweight* and *obesity* are meant to be used for documentation and risk assessment. More neutral terms such as *weight, excess weight, increased weight gain,* and *BMI* are to be used with families.
- Improvement in medical conditions is possible with changes in lifestyle habits, regardless of weight change.
- Patients can begin at the least intensive stage and advance depending on response to treatment, age, degree of obesity, health risks, and motivation.
- When a patient's habits, medical condition, weight, or BMI percentile do not improve in 3–6 months of planned treatment, the provider and family should consider advancing to the next, more intensive stage of treatment.
- Use motivational interviewing techniques to encourage the patient and family to set goals.

- Initial goals should be easily achievable.
- Use positive reinforcement.
- Focus on success, not failures.

References

Barlow S. Expert committee recommendations regarding the prevention, assessment and treatment of child and adolescent overweight and obesity: summary report. *Pediatrics.* 2007;120(4 Suppl):S164–S192.

Birch LL, Fisher JO. Development of eating behaviors among children and adolescents. *Pediatrics.* 1998;101(3 Pt 2):539–549.

Dubois L, Farmer A, Girard M, Peterson K. Regular sugar-sweetened beverage consumption between meals increases risk of overweight among preschool-aged children. *J Am Diet Assoc.* 2007;107(6):924–934.

Gillman MW, Rifas-Shiman SL, Frazier AL, et al. Family dinner and diet quality among older children and adolescents. *Arch Fam Med.* 2000;9(3):235–240.

Neumark-Sztainer D, Hannan PJ, Story M, Croll J, Perry C. Family meal patterns: associations with sociodemographic characteristics and improved dietary intake among adolescents. *J Am Diet Assoc.* 2003;103(3):317–322.

Nicklas TA, Morales M, Linares A, et al. Children's meal patterns have changed over a 21-year period: the Bogalusa Heart Study. *J Am Diet Assoc.* 2004;104(5):753–761.

Rampersaud GC, Pereira MA, Girard BL, Adams J, Metzl JD. Breakfast habits, nutritional status, body weight and academic performance in children and adolescents. *J Am Diet Assoc.* 2005;105(5):743–760.

Chapter 9
Pulmonary

Nutritional Algorithm for Bronchopulmonary Dysplasia/Chronic Lung Disease (BPD/CLD)

Bronchopulmonary Dysplasia/Chronic Lung Disease (BPD/CLD)

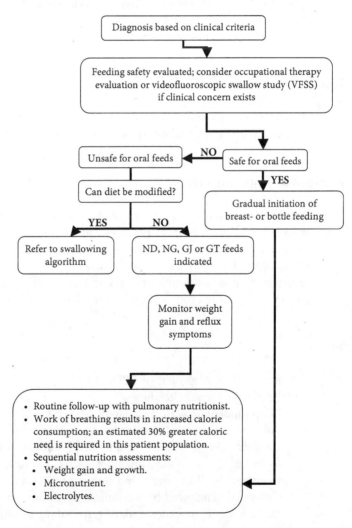

Pediatric Nutrition Handbook: An Algorithmic Approach, First Edition. Edited by David L. Suskind and Polly Lenssen.
© 2011 Blackwell Publishing Ltd. Published 2011 by Blackwell Publishing Ltd.

9.1   Bronchopulmonary Dysplasia/Chronic Lung Disease
Susan Casey

9.1.1   Name of Disorder

Bronchopulmonary dysplasia/chronic lung disease (BPD/CLD).

9.1.2   Clinical Definition

BPD/CLD is the result of injury to the developing lung by mechanical injury, oxygen toxicity, and infection, which results in pulmonary inflammation and damage. It includes a number of disorders involving the upper and lower respiratory tract. Bronchopulmonary dysplasia (BPD) is one form of chronic lung disease described in premature infants who may require mechanical ventilation and high concentrations of oxygen after birth.

9.1.3   How It Is Diagnosed

Premature infants and oxygen requirement at 28 days of life at 36 weeks postconceptual age, with radiographic abnormalities consistent with diagnosis.

9.1.4   Nutritional Implications

Patients may have one or more of the following, which may change caloric requirements: increased respiration rate, chronic low oxygen saturations, chronic or acute intercurrent illness or infection, growth failure from systemic corticosteroid therapy, gastroesophageal reflux (GER), fluid sensitivity, or other nutrition-related issues concurrent with prematurity, including necrotizing enterocolitis, central nervous system changes, and other delays.

9.1.5   Pearls

- Nutritional management of BPD/CLD:
  - Breast- or formula feeding.
  - Nasoduodenal (ND), nasogastric (NG), G-tube or G-tube feedings with bolus of continuous drip feeds, depending on the type and placement of the tube. (Most of these infants are gradually transitioned to some oral feeds based on swallowing safety after a stabilization period of several months as well as family and nursing training.)
  - Calorically enhanced breast milk, premature infant formula, and elemental formula as well as standard-term infant formula when appropriate.
  - Nonnutritive oral stimulation as well as feeding therapy is initiated through speech pathology and occupational therapy/physical therapy.

- Common medications that may affect nutrition:
  - Diuretics can cause increased micronutrient loss (e.g., furosemide causes calcium loss).
  - Bronchodilators.
  - Sedation medications.
  - Steroids.
- Medical complications affecting nutrition:
  - Fluid sensitivity requires increased caloric density to meet estimated caloric and protein needs.
  - GER with possible ascending aspiration requires continuous drip feeds.
  - Decreased oxygen saturations during oral or bolus feeds require supplemental oxygen during feeds.
  - Immature sucking, swallowing, and breathing patterns cause an increased risk of aspiration.
  - Descending aspiration requires thickened viscosity of feeds or tube feeding (i.e., NG or gastrostomy).
- Nutrients of concern:
  - Calories.
  - Protein.
  - Vitamins A and E.
  - Electrolytes.
  - Minerals.
  - Vitamin D, especially with lack of sun exposure.
- All nutritional assessments and recommendations are made on corrected age versus chronological age (e.g., a 12-month-old 28-week child is assessed as a 9-month-old). Recommendations for initiation of solid foods are also based on corrected age.

References

Kotecha S. Chronic respiratory complications of prematurity. In: Taussig LM, Landau LI, eds. *Pediatric Respiratory Medicine*. 2nd ed. St. Louis, MO: Mosby; 1999.

Wooldridge NH. Pulmonary diseases. In: Samour PQ, King K, eds. *Handbook of Pediatric Nutrition*. 3rd ed. Sudbury, MA: Jones and Bartlett; 2005.

Nutritional Algorithm for Cystic Fibrosis (CF)

Cystic Fibrosis (CF)

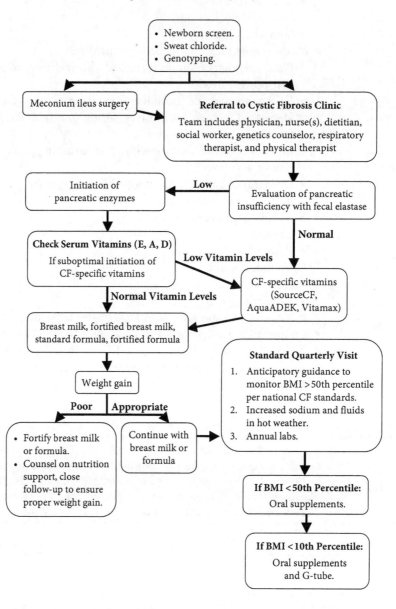

9.2   Cystic Fibrosis
Susan Casey

9.2.1   Name of Disorder

Cystic fibrosis (CF).

9.2.2   Clinical Definition

An autosomal, recessively inherited genetic disorder caused by mutations in the gene that encodes for the CF transmembrane regulator.

9.2.3   How It Is Diagnosed

CF newborn screening is now available throughout the entire continental United States. It consists of either immunoreactive trypsinogen (IRT) at birth, which is repeated 10 days afterward if the results are abnormal (the method in Washington state) or else IRT at birth and DNA testing if the IRT is abnormal (used in other states). All positive IRT/IRT or IRT/DNA results are followed by a sweat chloride test performed at an accredited lab for sweat tests.

9.2.4   Nutritional Implications

- Pancreatic insufficiency (malabsorption).
- Malnutrition.
- Chronic infections in the lungs resulting in increased metabolism.
- Increased metabolism due to the genetic defect.
- Pancreatitis (more common in pancreatic-sufficient patients).
- Distal intestinal obstruction syndrome.
- Meconium ileus.
- Chronic liver disease.
- CF-related diabetes.
- Hyponatremia.

9.2.5   Pearls

- There are 117 pediatric cystic fibrosis centers in the United States. The incidence of CF is 1 in 2500–3200 whites, 1 in 15,000 in African Americans. It is also seen in Asian and Native American populations at a much lower incidence.
- Nutrition goal: Goal is for weight gain and growth to be normal (to the child's genetic potential).
- Pancreatic insufficiency:

- 85% of patients have pancreatic insufficiency definitively diagnosed with a fecal elastase study. The symptoms include large, bulky, foul-smelling stools; poor weight gain despite a seemingly voracious appetite; excess flatulence; rectal prolapse and distal intestinal obstruction syndrome.
- Therapy consists of ingesting pancreatic enzymes in the form of capsules containing enteric-coated microspheres. These capsules are either swallowed whole or opened and the beads mixed in an acidic food such as fruit. The beads cannot be crushed or mixed in alkaline foods such as pudding or milk. Some microspheres are small enough to go through a small NG tube or gastrostomy tube (carefully).
- The Cystic Fibrosis Foundation recommends the amount of lipase (in kg/meal) not to exceed 2500 IU.
- Patients with pancreatic insufficiency may also malabsorb fat-soluble vitamins (such as A,D, E, and K). Vitamin levels are drawn at diagnosis and annually. CF-specific vitamins with a water-miscible form of fat-soluble vitamins are prescribed as liquid pediatric drops, chewable forms, and softgels.
- Caloric requirements: 130–150% of the Recommended Dietary Allowances (RDA) or Dietary Reference Intakes (DRI).
- Protein requirements: 200% of the DRI or RDA.
- CF -related diabetes:
  - Monitor clinical symptoms.
  - Oral Glucose Tolerance Test (OGTT) at 10 years and every year from then on.
    - Refer to Endocrinology for abnormal OGTT.
    - Some patients may have impaired glucose tolerance with a normal fasting glucose and an abnormal postprandial.
    - The goal of nutritional management is to manage hyperglycemia without compromising standard CF nutrition goals of increased caloric density, protein, fat, and sodium.
- Bone health: People with CF have an increased risk for osteomalacia and osteopenia due to the malabsorption of vitamin D. Vitamin D levels below normal are treated with extra vitamin D in addition to the CF-specific vitamins.

Nutritional Algorithm for Asthma

Asthma

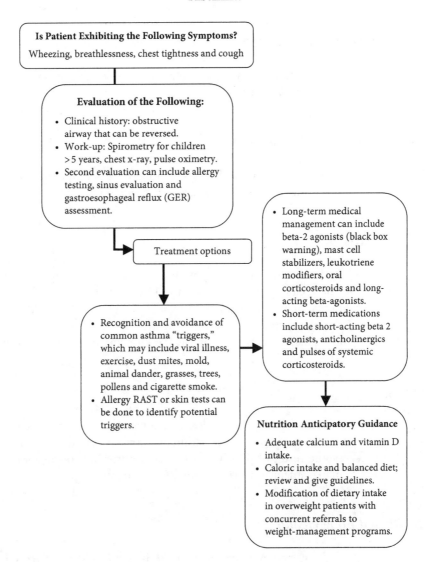

Is Patient Exhibiting the Following Symptoms?

Wheezing, breathlessness, chest tightness and cough

Evaluation of the Following:

- Clinical history: obstructive airway that can be reversed.
- Work-up: Spirometry for children >5 years, chest x-ray, pulse oximetry.
- Second evaluation can include allergy testing, sinus evaluation and gastroesophageal reflux (GER) assessment.

Treatment options

- Recognition and avoidance of common asthma "triggers," which may include viral illness, exercise, dust mites, mold, animal dander, grasses, trees, pollens and cigarette smoke.
- Allergy RAST or skin tests can be done to identify potential triggers.

- Long-term medical management can include beta-2 agonists (black box warning), mast cell stabilizers, leukotriene modifiers, oral corticosteroids and long-acting beta-agonists.
- Short-term medications include short-acting beta 2 agonists, anticholinergics and pulses of systemic corticosteroids.

Nutrition Anticipatory Guidance

- Adequate calcium and vitamin D intake.
- Caloric intake and balanced diet; review and give guidelines.
- Modification of dietary intake in overweight patients with concurrent referrals to weight-management programs.

9.3 Asthma

Susan Casey

9.3.1 Name of Disorder

Asthma.

9.3.2 Clinical Definition

A chronic inflammatory condition causing airway reversible obstruction.

9.3.3 How It Is Diagnosed

Clinical history and spirometry (reversible airway obstruction in response to bronchodilator trial).

9.3.4 Nutritional Implications

Some correlation with obesity; long-term steroid therapy may also result in bone mineral density and growth suppression.

9.3.5 Pearls

Asthma in the pediatric population has increased significantly since the 1980s. The incidence is greater in non-Hispanic blacks, children of lower socioeconomic status, African Americans, and males and children who have a first-degree relative with asthma. The most useful predictors are eczema as an infant and positive family history in the immediate family for asthma.

Obesity

Increased body mass index is associated with both a higher incidence and a marker for more severe asthma symptoms. In addition, obesity in asthma can be the result of poorly controlled symptoms. Caloric containment and weight management is a priority for these patients.

Growth and Bone Health

Chronic systemic steroid therapy is associated with growth suppression and decreased bone mineral density. Patients require a thorough review of dietary intake, particularly calcium and vitamin D, with recommendations for supplementation of both with a diet lacking in those nutrients or with prolonged steroid requirement.

Reference

Wooldridge NH. Pulmonary diseases. In: Samour PQ, King K, eds. *Handbook of Pediatric Nutrition*. 3rd ed. Sudbury, MA: Jones and Bartlett; 2005.

Chapter 10

Oncology

Nutritional Algorithm for Cancer

Cancer

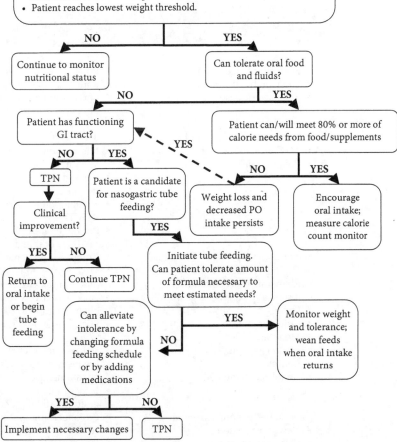

Pediatric Nutrition Handbook: An Algorithmic Approach, First Edition. Edited by David L. Suskind and Polly Lenssen.
© 2011 Blackwell Publishing Ltd. Published 2011 by Blackwell Publishing Ltd.

10.1   Cancer
Kathy Hunt

10.1.1   Name of Disorder

Cancer.

10.1.2   Nutritional Implications

Approximately 40–80% of children become malnourished during intensive cancer treatment. Malnutrition during chemotherapy is associated with increased infection rates, decreased tolerance of chemotherapy, delays in treatment, and diminished quality of life. Childhood cancers associated with the highest nutrition risk are presented in the table.

Childhood Cancer	Factors Affecting Nutritional Status
Wilms tumor • High risk: Stage III and IV • Unfavorable histology • Relapsed disease	• Surgical resection of tumor and kidney • Post-operative ileus. • Radiation therapy: younger patients often nothing per mouth (NPO) several hours prior to treatment
Neuroblastoma • High risk: Stage III and IV • *MYCN** amplification • Relapsed disease	• Young age (average age at diagnosis: 3.1 years) • Interruption in baseline feeding pattern • High need for enteral tube feeding • Postsurgery complications: High-output diarrhea • Hematopoietic stem cell transplantation (HSCT) • Prolonged transition after treatment back to 100% oral intake
Sarcomas • High risk: Stage III and IV • Rhabdomyosarcoma (RMS) (especially parameningeal RMS) • Ewing • Osteosarcoma • Metastatic disease Non-Hodgkin lymphoma • Burkitt • Anaplastic large cell	• Compressed chemotherapy cycles • Treatment with highly emetogenic and mucosal toxic chemotherapy • Lack of recovery time between chemotherapy to regain lost weight • High energy and protein requirements • Mucosal toxic chemotherapy • Frequent NPO status for intrathecal chemotherapy • Lack of interest in eating due to gastrointestinal mucosal damage
Acute myelogenous leukemia • Newly diagnosed • Relapsed disease	• Prolonged immunosuppression • At risk for fungal infections • Prolonged hospitalizations ("same old food" burnout)

Childhood Cancer	Factors Affecting Nutritional Status

Acute lymphocytic leukemia
High-risk categories:
• White blood cell count
  ≥50,000 mm³ and/or age ≥10 years
• Infants <12 months of age
• Chromosomal abnormalities:
  (Philadelphia+)
• T-cell phenotype
• Relapsed
Brain tumors
• Medulloblastoma and others
	• Need for cranial radiation
	• Treatment with highly emetogenic and
	  mucosal toxic chemotherapy
	• Asparaginase-induced pancreatitis
	• Steroid-induced hyperglycemia requiring
	  insulin
	• Frequent NPO status for procedures and
	  intrathecal chemotherapy
	• HSCT often necessary for cure
	• Treatment consists of 6 weeks of
	  radiation therapy
	• Younger children require sedation for
	  radiation (prolonged NPO status)
	• Hypogeusia
	• Nausea, vomiting, fatigue
	• Increased risk for dysphagia

*MYCN is an oncogene present on chromosome 2. The *MYCN* gene is amplified (has >10 copies instead of 2 copies) in a subset of neuroblastoma tumors; the amplification of the *MYCN* gene is associated with poor outcome.

10.1.3 Nutrition Intervention Goals

- Prevent or reverse nutritional deficits.
- Promote normal growth and development.
- Maximize quality of life.

It can be anticipated that the child undergoing cancer treatment will likely develop side effects (see later) that may prevent adequate calorie intake to maintain or restore nutritional status. Additionally, some chemotherapies are nephrotoxic and may cause increased losses of certain nutrients. For example, cisplatin commonly causes potassium, magnesium, calcium, and phosphorus wasting. Children receiving cancer treatment with nephrotoxic chemotherapy agents may require long-term supplementation of these nutrients.

The most appropriate nutrition intervention must meet the nutritional needs of the child while providing the least invasive method of administration. Maintaining oral feeds during cancer treatment is the preferred method of feeding; however, if oral feeding is not possible or is inadequate to meet nutrient needs, tube feeding should be initiated. Patients are typically fed nutritionally complete formulas that require normal digestion and absorption within the gastrointestinal (GI) tract. Patients with abnormal digestive or absorptive function with diarrhea or persistent vomiting, or those having difficulty gaining weight on intact formulas, may require use of elemental formulas.

Nasogastric feeds are typically provided as a continuous infusion versus bolus feeds, or a combination of both. Although bolus feeding schedules may be more physiologic, continuous feeding schedules are better tolerated due to GI problems of nausea, vomiting, or diarrhea.

10.1.4   Common Side Effects of Cancer Treatment Chemotherapy

- Nausea and vomiting.
- Alterations in taste and smell.
- Mucositis and esophagitis.
- Diarrhea.
- Constipation.
- Anorexia.
- Early satiety.
- Steroid-induced hyperglycemia.
- Pancreatitis.

10.1.5   Pearls

Hematology/oncology indications for total parenteral nutrition: pancreatitis, typhlitis, pancolitis pneumatosis, grade 4 mucositis without nasogastric tube in place, intractable diarrhea, severe vomiting.

References

Barale KV, Charuhas PM. Oncology and hematopoietic cell transplantation. In: Queen PS, King K, eds. *Handbook of Pediatric Nutrition.* 3rd ed. Sudbury, MA: Jones and Bartlett; 2005.

Ladas EJ, Sacks N, Meacham L, et al. A multidisciplinary review of nutrition considerations in the pediatric oncology population: a perspective from Children's Oncology Group. *Nutr Clin Pract.* 2005;20(4):377–393.

Mauer AM, Burgess JB, Donaldson SS, et al. Special nutritional needs of children with malignancies: a review. *J Parenteral Enteral Nutr.* 1990;14(3):315–324.

Chapter 11
Neurodevelopment

Nutritional Algorithm for Neurodevelopmental Delay

Neurodevelopmental Delay

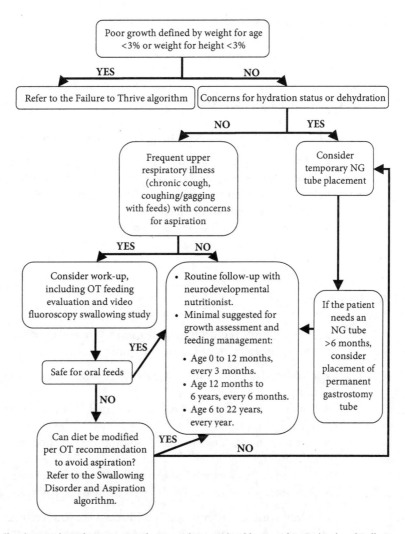

Pediatric Nutrition Handbook: An Algorithmic Approach, First Edition. Edited by David L. Suskind and Polly Lenssen.
© 2011 Blackwell Publishing Ltd. Published 2011 by Blackwell Publishing Ltd.

11.1   Neurodevelopmental Delay
Kim Cooperman

11.1.1   Name of Disorder

Feeding problems, including tube feedings in patients with neurodevelopmental delay.

11.1.2   Clinical Definition

Feeding disorders due to neurologic compromise.

11.1.3   How It Is Diagnosed

May present in many ways at any age.

11.1.4   Nutritional Implications

Children with neurodevelopmental delays are at increased risk for:

- Altered growth (i.e., underweight, overweight, short stature).
- Inadequate energy and nutrient intake to support growth and health.
- Feeding problems related to oral-motor and/or behavior difficulties.
- Need for enteral (tube) feeding.
- Chronic constipation or diarrhea.
- Gastroesophageal reflux.

11.1.5   Pearls

Signs/Symptoms requiring consideration of nasogastric, nasoduodenal, and gastrostomy feedings reported by the family:

- Prolonged feeding times. Meals take longer than an hour or total feeding time per day >4–6 hours.
- Frustration with feeding/eating so it is no longer a positive way to interact with the child.
- Stopping meals due to child choking, crying, and/or coughing as signs of discomfort.
- Hearing a "wet cough" associated with feeding/eating.
- Retching, vomiting, or other signs of distress with feeding or eating.

Children with low energy needs and receiving low volumes of tube feeding are at risk for inadequate intake of several nutrients, especially calcium, phosphorus, magnesium, protein, iron, and selenium as well as many vitamins.

11.1.6   Feeding Management

General Goals

1. Optimize oral intake and supplement with tube feeding.
2. Feeding regimen and formula are well-tolerated, that is, no gastrointestinal disturbance or other signs/symptoms of intolerance, and fits with family goals, preferences, and lifestyle (family-centered care).
3. Appropriate weight gain and growth.
4. Optimal nutrition (macro- and micronutrients) and hydration.
5. Consideration: Insurance/finances may impose limitations.

11.1.7   Common Problems with Tube Feeds

1. **Allergy:**
   - Change ingredients.
   - Change to elemental formula.
2. **Diarrhea:**
   - Malabsorption: Adjust ingredients.
   - Dumping: Slow feeding or if hyperosmolar, dilute formula.
3. **Gas:** Trial elemental formula or reduce/eliminate fiber.
4. **Gastroesophageal reflux disease:**
   - Concentrate formula to decrease volume.
   - Change feeding schedule to smaller bolus, slower bolus, or drip feedings.
   - Change position of tube, such as nasoduodenal or gastrojejunostomy.
     - Challenge: Maintaining hydration; plain water may be better tolerated.
5. **Constipation:**
   - Consider stool softeners such as polyethylene glycol.
   - Add fiber to formula or change to formula with fiber.
   - Assure adequate hydration.
6. **Overweight:**
   - Reduce caloric intake while maintaining hydration.
     - Challenge: Providing adequate vitamins and minerals and electrolytes.
7. **Underweight:**
   - Increase calories:
     - Increase volume.
     - Increase caloric density.
     - Add calorie boosters (such as Polycose, Duocal, Microlipid).

Chapter 12

Neonatology

Nutritional Algorithm for Feeding Infants in the NICU

Feeding Infants in the NICU

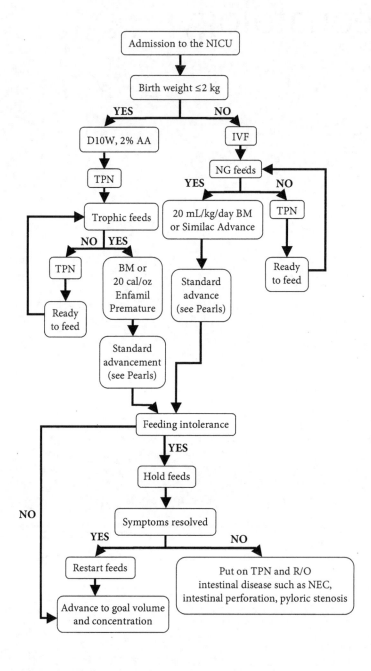

12.1   Feeding Infants in the Neonatal Intensive Care Unit

Maura Sandrock

The neonatal intensive care unit (NICU) admits infants ≤44 weeks term and preterm infants (adjusted age for preterm infants) with respiratory distress and congenital defects, including gastroschisis, omphalocele, diaphragmatic hernia, and congenital cardiac defects. Nutrition management and the nutrition plan are discussed on daily medical teams.

12.1.1   Pearls

Fluids

- Newborns: Fluids start with D10W at ~60–80 mL/g per day.
- Preterm infants: ≤2 kg, use D10W, 2.2% amino acids.
- Total fluids may be advanced by 20 mL/kg per day to fluids of 150–160 mL/kg.
- Fluid restriction (<140 mL/kg per day) is necessary for:
  - Congestive heart failure, patent ductus arteriosus (PDA), and other cardiac defects.
  - Diaphragmatic hernia.
  - Acute and chronic lung disease.
  - Surgery.
  - Renal insufficiency/failure.
- Increased fluid requirements can occur with:
  - Phototherapy.
  - Excess fluid losses, (i.e., unrepaired gastroschisis).
  - Nasogastric output.
  - Jejunostomy, ileostomy, or colostomy output.
  - Diarrhea.
  - Excessive urine output.
  - Very low birthweight.

Nutrition Support

- Trophic feeds are between 5 and 20 mL/kg per day; the initial feed volume is based on the infant's size and underlying gastrointestinal disease.
- In general, advancement of the feeds are between 15 and 30 mL/kg per day based on the infant's size and feeding tolerance.
- The concentration is increased to 22 cal/oz when at half the total volume of the feeds and to 24 cal/oz when at full volume.
- Advances of concentration >24 cal/oz by 2 cal/oz every 24–48 hours.
- Iron supplement 2–4 mg/kg per day when at full feeding.
- Poly-Vi-Sol multivitamin 1 mL daily for 100% breast-milk-fed babies not on human milk fortifier.

- Clinical signs of feeding intolerance (and possible concern for necrotizing enterocolitis [NEC]):
  - Residuals >3 mL/kg or >2-hour volume of feeds, whichever is larger. On trophic feeds, feeds should not be held for residual volumes <3 mL/kg.
  - Abdominal distention (>2 cm increase in girth), discoloration (red or blue), or tenderness.
  - Dark green residuals.
  - Frank blood or currant jelly in stools.
  - Pneumatosis on x-ray.
- Infants with a short small bowel due to NEC require a slow feeding advancement of 1–5 mL/kg per day.
- Advancement frequency is determined by stool output, clinical examination of abdomen, and underlying gastrointestinal disease.
- Hold the advances if the stool output is 30–35 mL/kg in 24 hours.
- Infants with birthweights <1.8 kg should transition from human milk fortifier or preterm formula to either NeoSure or Similac at the weight of ~2.5 kg.

Chapter 13

Nutrition Support

13.1   Enteral Nutrition

Polly Lenssen

Indications	Associated Conditions

Oral motor dysfunction or dysphagia	• Birth defects
	  • Esophageal atresia
	  • Tracheoesophageal fistula
	  • Pierre Robin syndrome
	• Brain tumors
	• Descending aspiration by videofluoroscopic swallow study (VFSS)
	• Neurologic disorders
	  • Cerebral palsy
	  • Cranial nerve dysfunction
	  • Muscular dystrophy
	  • Guillain-Barré syndrome
	  • Head injury/coma
	  • Myasthenia gravis

Increased metabolic needs	• Prematurity (<34 weeks) • Bronchopulmonary dysplasia • Burns • Congenital heart disease • Cystic fibrosis • Sepsis • Trauma • Wounds

Pediatric Nutrition Handbook: An Algorithmic Approach, First Edition. Edited by David L. Suskind and Polly Lenssen.
© 2011 Blackwell Publishing Ltd. Published 2011 by Blackwell Publishing Ltd.

Indications	Associated Conditions
Anorexia: Inadequate oral intake	• Cancer: leukemia, sarcoma, neuroblastoma, stem cell transplantation • FTT • Liver disease • Renal disease
Psychosocial disorders Malabsorption: Altered metabolism and/or other increased caloric loss	• Anorexia nervosa • Crohn's disease • Cystic fibrosis • Eosinophilic gastroenteritis • Glycogen storage disease (type 1 and 2) • Gastroesophageal reflux • Liver failure • Pseudo-obstruction • Pancreatitis • Short bowel syndrome
Increased length of time feeding (>4–6 hours per day)	• Batten disease • Cerebral palsy • Rett syndrome

13.1.1   When to Intervene with Enteral Nutrition

- Nutrient intake (energy, protein, fluid) are <75% estimated needs with concurrent weight loss.
- Child has failed trials of nutrient-dense oral supplements.
- Decrease in weight velocity (malnutrition) crosses two weight channels.
- Decrease in height velocity (stunting).
- Diminished muscle and/or fat reserves results in upper arm anthropometry <5th percentile.
- Dysphasia in NPO status.
- Therapies when expected outcome is anorexia, poor oral intake, and malnutrition without nutrition support (e.g., intensive cycles of chemotherapy).
- Weight reaches ≤90% ideal weight despite aggressive oral intervention.

13.1.2   Seattle Children's Enteral Formulary

There are market equivalents to most formulas; below are listed examples of what is required to have a complete formulary. Closed system is ideal in the hospital setting; pediatric products available in both open and closed systems are starred (*).

Premature

- Premature formula: Enfamil Premature.
- Breast milk + Similac HMF (human milk fortifier).
- Postpremature: NeoSure.

Infants

- Breast milk (can concentrate nutrient density with infant formulas and/or modular products).
- Standard infant formulas with iron: Similac.
- Soy infant formula: Isomil.
- Hydrolyzed protein: Alimentum, Nutramigen.
- Elemental formula: EleCare Infant.

Children 1–10 Years

- Standard pediatric formulas: Nutren Jr*, Nutren Jr with Fiber*, Compleat Pediatric, Bright Beginnings (soy).
- Semi-elemental/elemental formulas: Peptamen Jr*, Peptamen Jr with Fiber*, Peptamen Jr 1.5*, Vivonex Pediatric, Elecare Jr.

Children >10 Years

- Standard adult formulas: Osmolite*, Isosource HN* (soy).
- Fiber formulas: Compleat*, FiberSource HN* (soy).
- Semi-elemental/elemental: Peptamen*, Vivonex T.E.N.
- High calorie: Nutren 2*.

Modular Products

- Protein: Beneprotein.
- Carbohydrate: Polycose.
- Fat: Microlipid.
- Carbohydrate + fat: Duocal.
- Fiber: Nutrisource Fiber.

Specialty Products

- Renal failure, ketogenic, metabolic, critical care: Consult a dietitian.

Length of Therapy	Route	Tube Type/Size
Short term	Nasogastric Nasoduodenal • Indicated if severe reflux, emesis • Feeds must be given as continuous drip Nasojejunal • Placed by Interventional Radiology under fluoroscopy.	• Infants: 5–6 F • Children and adolescents: 6–8 F • Corpak or Frederick-Miller (only 8F, 70-cm, 110-cm length) • Frederick-Miller

Length of Therapy	Route	Tube Type/Size
Long term(>3 months)	Gastrostomy: Surgical Placement • Order surgery consult for evaluation of tube placement. • Requires 2-day admission or longer. • Not generally used until 7 days after placement to allow healing of tract; NG feeds required in interim. • Surgery available to follow up with problems	• Bard Button
	Gastrostomy: Endoscopic Placement (PEG) • Order GI consult for evaluation of tube placement • Requires 2-day admission • May be used within 24 hours after placement	• PEG tube: May be changed to MIC-KEY 12 weeks after placement; requires second surgical procedure
Long term (>3 months)	Gastrostomy: Poke and Dilate Procedure • Schedule with interventional radiology • May be used within 24 hours after placement • No standard follow-up with tube problems	• Ross Corflo gastrostomy tube: May be changed to G-tube button 12 weeks after placement; second surgical procedure not required
	Jejunostomy • Indicated if severe GE reflux, chronic vomiting • May be placed by surgery or interventional radiology • G/J tube may be placed after G-tube site is healed	• Frederick-Miller

Delivery Method*	Requires Pump?	Infusion Schedule	Comments
*Based on tube type, quantity and concentration of formula, tolerance to formula and child/parent schedule.			
Continuous Drip Feeds • When initiating feeds • Small bowel feed • When other methods are not tolerated	Yes	Infused at a prescribed rate over 24 hours	Difficult to use for active children as being hooked up to the pump limits activity
Cyclic drip feeds	Yes	Infused over 8–18 hours	Allows time off pump
Bolus feeds Syringe • Least expensive	No	4–6 feeds/day given over 5–15 minutes or longer	Allows most normal schedule
Gravity Drip • Uses bag	No	3–5 feeds/day given over 20–45 minutes	
Intermittent with pump • When syringe feeding is not tolerated	Yes.	3–5 feeds/day given over 30–60 minutes	
Combination: Bolus and cyclic drip feeds • When unable to give all bolus feeds during day • When child is eating during day	Yes	Variable	

13.1.3   Initiation and Advancement of Feeds

Preterm

- Continuous: Initial 0.5–1 mL/kg/hr; advance 10–20 mL/kg/day to goal 120–175 mL/kg/day.
- Bolus: Initial 2–4 mL/kg/feed; advance 2–4 mL/feed to goal 120–175 mL/kg/day.

Infants

- Continuous: Initial 1–2 mL/kg/hr; advance 1–2 mL/kg every 2–8 hr to goal 6 mL/kg/hr.
- Bolus: Initial 10–15 mL/kg every 2–3 hr; advance 10–30 mL/feed to goal 20–30 mL/kg every 4–5 hr.

Children < 5 yr

- Continuous: Initial 1 mL/kg/hr; advance 1 mL/kg every 2–8 hr to goal 4–5 mL/kg/hr.
- Bolus: Initial 5–10 mL/kg every 3 hr; advance 30–45 mL/feed to goal 15–20 mL/kg every 4–5 hr.

Children > 5 yr

- Continuous: Initial 25–35 mL/hr; advance 25 mL/kg every 2–8 hr to estimated maintenance fluid needs.
- Bolus: Initial 90–120 mL every 3–4 hr; advance 60–90 mL/feed to goal 330–480 mL every 4–5 hr.

13.1.4   Extra Water

- Water flushes should be given after each bolus feed and when drip feeds are stopped for tube patency. It is best to order how much water to give as flushes.
- Additional water flushes may be needed throughout the day depending on total fluid needs.

13.1.5   Monitoring

- Emesis, diarrhea, bloating, and irritability are possible indicators of intolerance to feeding schedule or type of formula and/or concentration.
- Rapid weight gain and edema are possible indicators of overhydration.
- Decreased urination and constipation are possible indicators of underhydration.

13.1.6   Transition to Oral Feeds

- Does child need to work with occupational therapist?
- Does swallowing evaluation by speech therapy need to be done?
- A meal plan for implementing solid foods needs to be considered.
- Monitor oral intake with daily calorie counts initially.
- Oral intake should meet at least 75% of nutrient needs before discontinuing tube feeding.
- G-tubes should be left in place until it is evident that oral intake is adequate.

13.1.7   Discharging a Patient on Tube Feeding

- Ideally patient is tolerating full feeds.
- Allow 2 days for discharge planning, teaching, and supply delivery.
- Identify follow-up plan for patient with dietitian.

Nutritional Algorithm for TPN

13.2   Indications for Total Parenteral Nutrition
Polly Lenssen

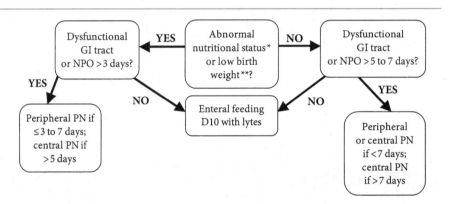

* *<5th percentile weight for age, weight for height, or body mass index for age.*
** *<2500 g.*
Adopted from Duggan et al., 2002.

13.2.1   Conditions Associated with Total Parenteral Nutrition

- Bowel rest for ≥5 days.
- Severe cardiac insufficiency.
- Chronic idiopathic intestinal pseudo-obstruction syndrome.
- Gastrointestinal fistulas.
- Inflammatory bowel disease (when failure to maintain growth and development occurs).
- Intractable diarrhea of infancy.

- Low birthweight infants.
- Malabsorption (severe).
- Marrow (myeloablative regimens) and organ transplantation.
- Chylothorax and chylous ascites.
- Short gut syndrome.

13.2.2   Nutrient Requirements

1. **Fluids:** See Chapter 1, "General Pediatric Nutrition Assessment" section.
2. **Energy:**
   a. Increased needs with high activity levels, stress, wounds, catch-up growth, or repletion.
   b. Decreased needs with bed rest, sedation, paralysis, and excess adiposity.

Age	kcal/kg/Day
Preterm	90–120
Term <6 months	85–105
6–12 months	80–100
1–7 years	75–90
7–12 years	50–75
12–18 years	30–35

3. **Fat:**
   a. 30–40% of total calories.
   b. Minimum amount to prevent essential fatty acid deficiency is 4–8% of total energy.
   c. Maximum amount is 60% of total calories and/or typically 3 g/kg.
   d. More than 1 g/kg in long-term TPN may contribute to cholestasis.
   e. Infusion rate should not exceed 0.15 g/kg per hour.

	g/kg/Day IV Lipids					
	Preterm	Term	6–12 Months	Toddlers	Children	Adolescents
Begin at	0.5	0.5	1	1	1	1
Advance daily as tolerated	0.5	0.5	0.5	0.5–1	0.5–1	0.5–1
Usual max	2.5–3	2–3	2–3	2–3	2–3	1.5–2

4. **Carbohydrate:**
   a. 40–50% of energy (3.4 kcal/g).
   b. Greater doses may lead to hyperglycemia, cholestasis, and fatty liver.

	mg/kg/Min Dextrose			g/Day		
	Preterm	Term	6–12 Months	Toddlers	Children	Adolescents
Begin at*	4–6	6–7	6–7	8–10	6–8	4–5
Advance daily as tolerated	2	2	2	2–3	2–3	2–3
Goal	10–12	12–14	12–14	18–20	12–15	7–10

5. **Protein:**
   a. 4 kcal/g.
   b. In patients with fluid restrictions and who are unable to receive adequate nutrition, protein needs should have priority.
   c. Children <12 months receive a pediatric amino acid formulation fortified with histidine, taurine, and tyrosine with added cysteine (conditionally essential in infants on TPN).

	g/kg/Day Protein					
	Preterm*	Term	6–12 Months	Toddlers	Children	Adolescents
Begin at	3	2	2	1–2	1–2	0.8–1.5
Advance daily as tolerated	1	1	1	1		
Goal	3–4	2–3	2–3	1–2	1–2	0.8–1.5

*Infants with gastroschisis: Start at 3 g/kg regardless of gestational age.

6. **Electrolytes:**

Electrolyte and Mineral Requirements			
	Preterm mEq/kg/Day	Term mEq/kg/Day	Toddlers/Children mEq/kg/Day (Ordered as mEq/Day)	Adolescents mEq/Day
Sodium	2–5	2–5	1–2	60–100
Potassium	2–4	2–4	1–2	70–150
Magnesium	0.3–0.5	0.3–0.5	0.3–0.5	10–30
Calcium	2–4 Mmol/kg/day	0.5–4 Mmol/kg/day	0.5–4 Mmol/kg/day	10–20 Mmol/kg/day
Phosphorus	1–2	0.5–2	0.5–2.0	10–40

Chloride and acetate: No specific requirement; add as needed to maintain acid base balance.

7. **Vitamins:**
   a. Provided by age and weight using a pediatric multivitamin (MVI) formulation for patients <11 years of age and an adult MVI formulation for patients ≥11 years of age.
   b. Patients on long-term TPN may require reduced MVI dosing based on serum levels.

Vitamin Requirements		
	<11 Years Old MVI Pediatric Dosing: 2 mL/kg (Maximum 5 mL)	≤11 Years Old MVI Adult (Multi-12) Dosing: 10 mL
Sodium	2–5	2–5

Vitamin	Content per 5 mL	Content per 10 mL
A	2300 IU	3300 IU
D	400 IU	200 IU
E	7 IU	10 IU
B$_1$ (thiamine)	1.2 mg	6 mg
B$_2$ (riboflavin)	1.4 mg	3.6 mg
B$_3$ (niacin)	17 mg	40 mg
K (phytonadione)	200 µg	150 µg
Pantothenic acid	5 mg	15 mg
B$_6$ (pyridoxine)	1 mg	6 mg
B$_{12}$ (cyanocobalamin)	1 µg	5 µg
Ascorbic acid	80 mg	200 mg
Biotin	20 µg	60 µg
Folic acid	140 µg	600 µg

8. **Trace elements:**

   Commercial trace element packages do not meet expert recommendations, and a trace element cocktail is compounded. Selenium and molybdenum are added after >30 days of TPN (selenium is added in neonates on day 1 of TPN).

	Trace Elements Requirements			
	Preterm Neonates <3 kg	**Term Neonates** 3–10 kg	**Children 10–40 kg**	**Adolescents** >40 kg
Chromium	0.05–0.2 µg/kg/day	0.2 µg/kg/day	0.14–0.2 µg/kg/day	5–15 µg
Copper	20 µg/kg/day	20 µg/kg/day	5–20 µg/kg/day	0.2–0.5 mg
Manganese	1 µg/kg/day	1 µg/kg/day	1 µg/kg/day	40–100 µg
Zinc	400 µg/kg/day	50–250 µg/kg/day	50–125 µg/kg/day	2–5 mg

   a. Iron: Not added to TPN due to solubility concerns.
   b. Carnitine: Essential for transport of fatty acids across the inner mitochondrial membrane into the mitochondrial matrix where the enzymes for beta oxidation are located. Premature infants have low reserves.
      - Preterm neonates: <2 kg: 10 mg/kg/day; 2 kg: 5 mg/kg/day.
      - Term infants NPO >2 weeks: 5 mg/kg/day.
   c. Zinc: To compensate for large stool or fistula losses, add 1 mg for every 100 mL stool above:
      - 250 mL stool in patients <20 kg.
      - 500 mL stool in patients 20–40 kg.
      - 1000 mL stool in patients >40 kg.

13.2.3 Aluminum Content of PN Solutions

Patients with impaired kidney function or premature neonates and patients on long-term TPN accumulate aluminum at levels associated with bone and central nervous system toxicity. Products highest in aluminum content (from highest to lowest): potassium phosphate, sodium phosphate, calcium gluconate, L-cysteine. In addition to products used in preparing PN, other sources of aluminum include heparin, albumin, and blood products.

13.2.4   Peripheral PN

- Indicated when central access is unavailable or for short-term use (at least >3 days).
- Maximum potassium content is 60 mEq/L and osmolality is 900 mOsm/L.
- Coadministration with lipids prolongs peripheral venous catheter life and protects against thrombophlebitis owing to the isotonicity of the lipid emulsion.

	Minimum Monitoring Guidelines for Safe TPN		
Variables (recommended)	**Metabolic Instability (first week or during metabolic instability)**	**Metabolic Steady State (first month/metabolically stable)**	**Long-Term TPN (>1 month/ metabolically stable)**
Electrolytes	Daily	Twice weekly (Mon., Thurs.)	Monthly
I-Ca, PO4, Mg	Daily	Weekly (Mon.)	Monthly
Glucose	Daily	Twice weekly (Mon, Thurs.)	Monthly
BUN, creatinine	Twice weekly (Mon., Thurs.)	Weekly (Mon.)	Monthly
Pre-albumin	Weekly (Mon)*	Monthly*	Every other month
Albumin	Weekly (Mon)	First of every month	Every other month
LFTs (ALT/AST/bilirubin [unconjugated/ conjugated])	Twice weekly (Mon., Thurs.)	Weekly (Mon.)	Every 3 months
Triglycerides	Daily* until goal is reached (except infants: See IICU Guidelines)	Weekly (Mon.)	Every 3 months
Hgb, Hct	Twice weekly (Mon., Thurs.)	Twice weekly (Mon., Thurs.)	Monthly
Trace elements (manganese, copper, chromium)			Every 6 months
Zinc			Monthly
Selenium			Every 3 months
Folate			Every 3 months
Vitamin A + retinol binding protein			Every 3 months
Vitamin D (25-OH)			Every 3 months
Vitamin E			Every 3 months
Prothrombin time			Every 3 months

13.2.5   Management of Metabolic Complications

Management of Metabolic Complications		
Complication	**Definition**	**Intervention**
Hyperglycemia ICU patients may require an insulin drip to control blood sugar more tightly	Serum glucose >180 mg/dL on two blood draws while on PN OR Serum glucose >180 mg/dL + capillary stick	1. Can dextrose or total calories be decreased? 2. Can lipid calories be substituted for dextrose calories? 3. If energy support is appropriate, starting dose is 1 unit of insulin for every 20 g of PN dextrose, and correction dose is based on glucose checks every 6 hours • 200–300 mg/dL: 0.04 units/kg • 301–400 mg/dL: 0.08 units/kg • 401–500 mg/dL: insulin drip Goal: Maintain serum glucose 100–180 mg/dL
Hypertriglyceridemia	Infants: >200–300 mg/dL Children >1 year: >300–400 mg/dL during infusion or >250 mg/dL 4 hours after lipid infusion	Decrease lipid dose by 50%
Hypertriglyceridemia (continued)	Infants: >300 mg/dL Children >1 year: >400 mg/dL	Infants: Hold lipids until triglyceride level normalizes Children: Provide lipids very conservatively to meet essential fatty acid requirements (4–6% total calories). Risk of pancreatitis increases when serum triglycerides >1000 mg/dL
TPN-induced cholestasis		1. Prevent overfeeding 2. Limit lipids to 1 g/kg/day 3. Reduce copper 50%; delete manganese when conjugated bilirubin >2 4. Start trophic, enteral feeds if possible 5. Maintain tight glucose control and triglycerides in normal range 6. Test serum carnitine and supplement as needed 7. Institute Omegaven if approved and consented
Refeeding syndrome (electrolytes and minerals shift from extracellular to intracellular space to support anabolism)	Low serum potassium, phosphorus and/or magnesium after initiation of PN	1. Progress PN to goal over several days 2. Check serum electrolytes and minerals daily during the progression of PN to goal 3. Provide bolus repletion doses of any low electrolytes and adjust PN doses upward
Hypoglycemia can develop rapidly with abrupt discontinuation of TPN	Blood sugar <60 mg/dL	1. A 1- to 2-hour taper may be needed to prevent rebound hyperglycemia 2. If a PN solution must be discontinued quickly, give D5 or D10 for at least 1 hour following discontinuation
Essential fatty acid deficiency	Triene: tetraene ratio >0.4.	1. Neonates: Give IV lipids as 4% to 5% of total calories 2. Older children: Give 0.5 g/kg standard lipids 3. Omegaven: Give 1 g/kg

TPN Modifications during Organ Failure			
	Protein	**Fat**	**Dextrose**	**Electrolytes, Vitamins and Trace Elements**
Liver	1 g/kg in presence of encephalopathy; pediatric amino acid solution	Limit to 1 g/kg with cholestasis		When conjugated bilirubin >2, reduce copper dose by 50% and remove manganese Test serum levels to avoid deficiency/toxicity
Renal	Restrict to half of estimated needs if BUN >80–100 mg/dL			Potassium, phosphate, calcium and magnesium are typically restricted; selenium and chromium may need to be reduced or eliminated in prolonged renal failure
CRRT	0.2 g/kg of protein should be added to compensate for losses across the filter		Serum glucose <140 mg/dL to minimize glucose losses across the filter	Renal replacement vitamins in addition to the standard MVI to compensate for large water-soluble losses via the filter After 1 week, assay serum vitamin A and retinol-binding protein (RBP) levels to calculate molar ratio of vitamin A to RBP
ECMO		Compatible with silicone membrane or Quadrox oxygenator or on CPS with a hollow fiber oxygenator		

*Sample renal replacement vitamin "cocktail":
Infants: Thiamine 0.7 mg, B12 0.25 mcg, Folic Acid 70 mcg, Vitamin C 100 mg.
Children 1-11 yr: Thiamine 25 mg, Riboflavin 0.5 mg, Niacin 25 mg, Pantothenic Acid 0.5 mg, Pyridoxine 15 mg, B12 15 mcg, Folic Acid 0.5 mg, Vitamin C 45 mg.
Children 11 yr and older: Thiamine 50 mg, Riboflavin 1 mg, Niacin 50 mg, Pantothenic Acid 1 mg, Pyridoxine 30 mg, B12 30 mcg, Folic Acid 1 mg, Vitamin C 90 mg.

References

American Academy of Pediatrics Committee on Nutrition. *Pediatric Nutrition Handbook*. 6th ed. Elk Grove Village, IL: American Academy of Pediatrics; 2009.

ASPEN Board of Directors and the Clinical Guidelines Task Force. Guidelines for the use of parenteral and enteral nutrition in adult and pediatric patients. *J Parenter Enteral Nutr.* 2002;26(1 Suppl):1SA–138SA.

ASPEN Nutrition Support Practice Manual, 2nd edition, 2005.

Duggan C, Rizzo C, Cooper A, et al. Effectiveness of a clinical practice guideline for parenteral nutrition: a 5-year follow-up study in a pediatric teaching hospital. *J Parenter Enteral Nutr.* 2002;26(6):377–381.

Mirtallo J, Canada T, Johnson D, et al; Task Force for the Revision of Safe Practices for Parenteral Nutrition. Safe practices for parenteral nutrition. *J Parenter Enteral Nutr.* 2004;28(6):S39–S70.

Chapter 14

Surgery

Nutritional Algorithm for Post-operative Nutritional Care

Post-operative Nutritional Care

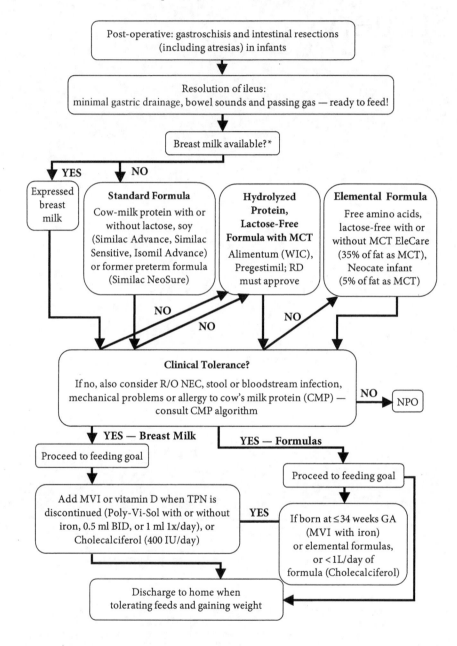

Post-operative: gastroschisis and intestinal resections (including atresias) in infants

Resolution of ileus:
minimal gastric drainage, bowel sounds and passing gas — ready to feed!

Breast milk available?*

YES **NO**

Expressed breast milk

Standard Formula
Cow-milk protein with or without lactose, soy (Similac Advance, Similac Sensitive, Isomil Advance) or former preterm formula (Similac NeoSure)

Hydrolyzed Protein, Lactose-Free Formula with MCT
Alimentum (WIC), Pregestimil; RD must approve

Elemental Formula
Free amino acids, lactose-free with or without MCT EleCare (35% of fat as MCT), Neocate infant (5% of fat as MCT)

NO **NO** **NO**

Clinical Tolerance?
If no, also consider R/O NEC, stool or bloodstream infection, mechanical problems or allergy to cow's milk protein (CMP) — consult CMP algorithm

NO → NPO

YES — Breast Milk

Proceed to feeding goal

YES — Formulas

Proceed to feeding goal

Add MVI or vitamin D when TPN is discontinued (Poly-Vi-Sol with or without iron, 0.5 ml BID, or 1 ml 1x/day), or Cholecalciferol (400 IU/day)

YES

If born at ≤34 weeks GA (MVI with iron) or elemental formulas, or <1L/day of formula (Cholecalciferol)

Discharge to home when tolerating feeds and gaining weight

*If infant is on specialized formula prior to surgery or has a significant bowel resection, may restart

If infant is on specialized formula before surgery or has a significant bowel resection, may restart presurgical/elemental formula.

Nutritional Algorithm for Oral/Enteral Feeding Advancement

Oral/Enteral Feeding Advancement

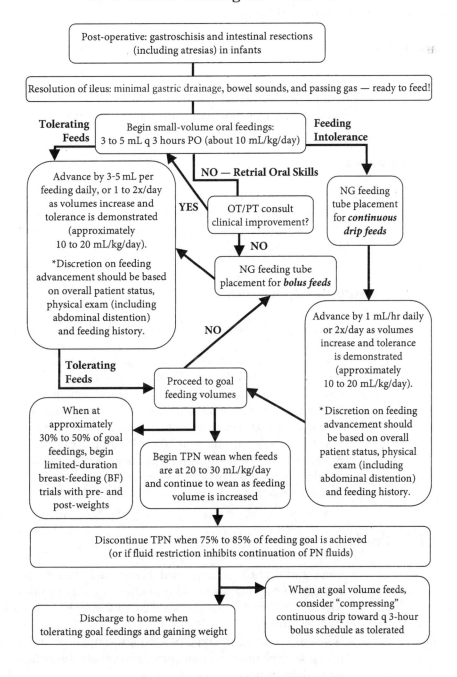

Post-operative: gastroschisis and intestinal resections (including atresias) in infants

Resolution of ileus: minimal gastric drainage, bowel sounds, and passing gas — ready to feed!

Begin small-volume oral feedings: 3 to 5 mL q 3 hours PO (about 10 mL/kg/day)

Tolerating Feeds

Feeding Intolerance

Advance by 3-5 mL per feeding daily, or 1 to 2x/day as volumes increase and tolerance is demonstrated (approximately 10 to 20 mL/kg/day).

*Discretion on feeding advancement should be based on overall patient status, physical exam (including abdominal distention) and feeding history.

NO — Retrial Oral Skills

OT/PT consult clinical improvement?

YES

NO

NG feeding tube placement for *continuous drip feeds*

NG feeding tube placement for *bolus feeds*

Advance by 1 mL/hr daily or 2x/day as volumes increase and tolerance is demonstrated (approximately 10 to 20 mL/kg/day).

*Discretion on feeding advancement should be based on overall patient status, physical exam (including abdominal distention) and feeding history.

Tolerating Feeds

NO

Proceed to goal feeding volumes

When at approximately 30% to 50% of goal feedings, begin limited-duration breast-feeding (BF) trials with pre- and post-weights

Begin TPN wean when feeds are at 20 to 30 mL/kg/day and continue to wean as feeding volume is increased

Discontinue TPN when 75% to 85% of feeding goal is achieved (or if fluid restriction inhibits continuation of PN fluids)

When at goal volume feeds, consider "compressing" continuous drip toward q 3-hour bolus schedule as tolerated

Discharge to home when tolerating goal feedings and gaining weight

14.1   Post-operative Nutritional Care
Jenny Stevens

14.1.1   General Surgical Diagnoses

Gastroschisis

Ventral/abdominal wall defect, where the bowel is extended freely in the amniotic fluid space through an opening usually to the right of the umbilicus. Diagnosis is made on prenatal ultrasound or at birth.

Intestinal atresia

Failure of a portion of the intestine to completely form, causing an absence or closure of a part of the intestine. Diagnosis is made on prenatal ultrasound or shortly after birth, presenting as feeding intolerance resulting in abdominal distention, failure to pass stool, and emesis with feedings.

14.1.2   Nutritional Implications

- Variable malabsorption of enteral nutrients and energy, potentially impacting growth and development.
- Potential need for specialty infant formulas, an alternative route of feeding due to intolerance of oral/gastric feedings, and/or oral feeding aversion related to delayed initiation of oral feedings or negative stimulus from vomiting.
- Prolonged total parenteral nutrition (TPN) use increases risk of liver disease.
- Potential anemia related to preterm delivery/birth, chronic blood draws, and iron-free parenteral nutrition (PN) (IV iron is cautiously used), as well as prolonged time before full feedings are achieved, and/or before enteral iron supplementation is provided or tolerated.
- Increased risk for necrotizing enterocolitis (NEC).

14.1.3   Pearls

- Limit fortification of expressed breast milk (EBM) or concentration of formula to patients with fluid restrictions or volume intolerance.
- Risk of NEC may increase with increased osmolality from fortifying breast milk or formula.
- When determining the type of specialty formula to use, consider length of resection, type of bowel remaining, and expected substrate to be of concern for malabsorption.
- Test stool for malabsorption:
  a. Carbohydrate (mainly lactose): Increased stool-reducing substances.
  b. Fat: Increased free/neutral fecal fat.

- If patient fails to gain weight on sufficient energy/protein intake, consider checking serum and urine sodium; may need sodium chloride (NaCl) supplementation.
- With significant malabsorption, the patient may need additional supplementation of vitamins and minerals.
  a. With significant fat malabsorption, use a water-miscible vitamin preparation (SourceCF or ADEK 1 mL/day).
  b. Check vitamin levels as needed.
- Hypo-osmolar feedings (15–19 kcal/oz formula) may be used in extreme malabsorption (usually applies to elemental formulas).
- Consult occupational therapist/physical therapist (OT/PT) at any point to evaluate oral feeding skills and assist with breast-feeding or any other oral feeding-related or lactation-related concerns.
- Trial breast-feeding or small oral-binky-training feedings may begin at any point, and as determined safe and appropriate by the surgical team, in consultation with OT/PT.
- For mothers intending to breast-feed, encourage pumping to maintain a production of ≥20 oz/day.
- For tube-fed patients on an every-3-hour feeding schedule, the gravity bolus regimen is preferred over the pump-assisted longer duration bolus regimen to minimize equipment needs.
- On goal feedings, 1–2 days of weight gain is preferable (20–40 g/day for infants 0–4 months) prior to discharge.

Chapter 15

Intensive Care: Cardiac/Pediatric

Nutritional Algorithm for Chylothorax

Chylothorax

```
                            ┌─────────────────────┐
                            │    Chylothorax      │
                            └─────────────────────┘
                                       │
                                       ▼
                            ┌─────────────────────────┐
                            │ • NPO x 24 hr.          │
                            │ • Determine baseline    │
                            │   chyle output before   │
                            │   initiating.           │
                            │ • Nutrition support.    │
                            │ • D5-10% to IV support. │
                            └─────────────────────────┘
```

┌──────────────────┐   ┌──────────────────┐
│ TPN, including   │   NO   │ Able to tolerate │
│ lipids, until   │ ◄─────── │ enteral feeds   │
│ enteral feeds can│   └──────────────────┘
│ be started   │   │
└──────────────────┘   **YES**

┌──────────────────┐
│ Able to tolerate │ ──── **NO** ────►
│   oral feeds   │
└──────────────────┘
        │
      YES

┌────────────────────────────────────┐   ┌──────────────────┐
│ • Fat-free or low-fat diet   │   │ • Nasogastric or │
│   supplemented with MCT oil   │   │   nasoduodenal   │
│   OR   │   │   feeds.   │
│ • Lipistart high-MCT formula   │   │ • Lipistart   │
│   x 24 hours.   │   │   high-MCT   │
│   │   │   formula   │
│   │   │   x 24 hours.   │
└────────────────────────────────────┘   └──────────────────┘

┌──────────────────────┐
│ Reassess chylos leak│
└──────────────────────┘

┌──────────────────┐   ┌──────────────────┐
│ ↑ Chylos output │   │ ↓ Chylos output │
└──────────────────┘   └──────────────────┘

┌──────────────────┐   ┌────────────────────────────┐
│ Start TPN and IV │   │ • Continue enteral feeds. │
│ lipids x 3 days │   │   OR   │
└──────────────────┘   │ • Restart enteral feeds   │
                              │   if receiving TPN.   │
                              └────────────────────────────┘

Pediatric Nutrition Handbook: An Algorithmic Approach, First Edition. Edited by David L. Suskind and Polly Lenssen.
© 2011 Blackwell Publishing Ltd. Published 2011 by Blackwell Publishing Ltd.

15.1   Chylothorax

Claudia Sassano-Miguel

15.1.1   Name of Disorder

Chylothorax.

15.1.2   Clinical Definition

Chyle leakage occurs as a result of lymphatic injury from trauma or surgery in the chest, abdomen, or neck.

15.1.3   How It Is Diagnosed

Observed chylous drainage from a chest or other drainage tube. Fluid containing >100 mg/dL of triglycerides is considered indicative of a chyle leak.

15.1.4   Nutritional Implications

Decrease the production of chyle fluid by restricting long-chain triglycerides while maintaining or repleting nutritional status.

15.1.5   Pearls

Parenteral lipids are phospholipids delivered directly into the bloodstream and as a result do not pass through the lymph system as chyle. Therefore, IV lipids are *not* contraindicated in patients with chyle leaks.

Nutritional Algorithm for Patients on Extracorporeal Membrane Oxygenation (ECMO)

Patients on Extracorporeal Membrane Oxygenation (ECMO)

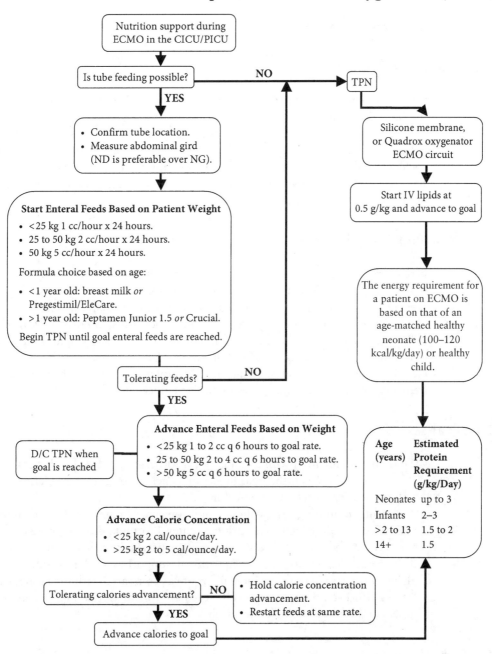

15.2   Extracorporeal Membrane Oxygenation
Claudia Sassano-Miguel

15.2.1   Name of Disorder

Extracorporeal membrane oxygenation (ECMO).

15.2.2   Clinical Definition

Extracorporeal life support (ECLS) or extracorporeal membrane oxygenation (ECMO) use a cardiopulmonary bypass circuit for temporary life support for patients with potentially reversible life-threatening cardiac and/or pulmonary failure. Common diagnoses using ECLS/ECMO include pneumonia, sepsis, persistent pulmonary hypertension, acute lung injury, acute respiratory distress syndrome, post-operative cardiac surgery, and end-stage cardiac disease as a bridge to transplantation.

15.2.3   Nutritional Implications

Patients receiving ECLS/ECMO may demonstrate significant lean muscle catabolism that places them at risk for protein malnutrition associated with loss of skeletal muscle, need for a prolonged mechanical ventilation, and even the compromise of long-term developmental outcomes. Most children who receive ECLS/ECMO now survive the acute illness but often sustain significant long-term morbidity, including feeding difficulties. These nutritional problems may include incoordination of sucking and swallowing, gastroesophageal reflux, frequent regurgitation, and delays in gastric emptying.

15.2.4   Pearls

- Start enteral nutrition with formula of caloric density, 30 kcal/oz for children >1 year of age. When the goal fluid rate is achieved, gradually increase the caloric density to achieve goal calories.
- Frequently monitor gastric volumes and stop enteral nutrition if gastric retention occurs. Following the cessation of enteral formula delivery, hold enteral feeds for 24 hours and then reinitiate if the patient remains stable.
- In general, delivery of enteral nutritional support is probably safer when delivery occurs via the nasoduodenal route as compared with the nasogastric route. However, if nasogastric tube feeds are tolerated, this more likely represents a more physiologic approach.

Reference

Jaksic T, et al. ASPEN Clinical Guidelines: Nutrition Supported with Extracorporeal Membrane Oxygenation. *J Parenteral Enteral Nutr.* 2010;34(3).

Chapter 16
Cardiology

Nutritional Algorithm for Congenital Heart Disease

Congenital Heart Disease

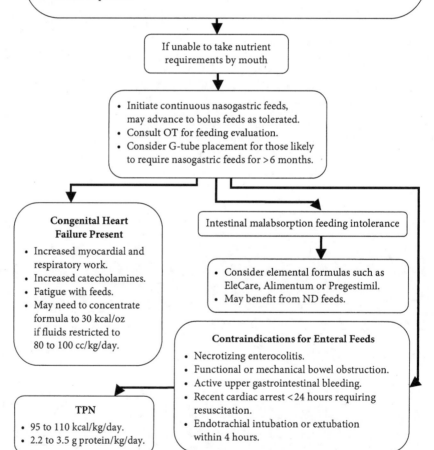

Undernutrition in Congenital Heart Disease (CHD) Nutrition Assessment

- Type of CHD.
- Anthropometric measurements: weight, height, occipital frontal circumference.
- Feeding pattern, ability to feed PO, medications.
- Diet management should always be done in conjunction with the cardiology team.
- Labs: lytes, calcium phosphorus, albumin, pre-albumin, hemocrit, hemoglobin, socioeconomic factors.

General Nutrient Requirements

- 120 to160 kcal/kg/day.
- 2.5 to 3.5 g protein/kg/day.
- 35% to 60% carbohydrate.
- 35% to 50% fat.
- 8% to 10% protein.

If unable to take nutrient requirements by mouth

- Initiate continuous nasogastric feeds, may advance to bolus feeds as tolerated.
- Consult OT for feeding evaluation.
- Consider G-tube placement for those likely to require nasogastric feeds for >6 months.

Congenital Heart Failure Present

- Increased myocardial and respiratory work.
- Increased catecholamines.
- Fatigue with feeds.
- May need to concentrate formula to 30 kcal/oz if fluids restricted to 80 to 100 cc/kg/day.

Intestinal malabsorption feeding intolerance

- Consider elemental formulas such as EleCare, Alimentum or Pregestimil.
- May benefit from ND feeds.

Contraindications for Enteral Feeds

- Necrotizing enterocolitis.
- Functional or mechanical bowel obstruction.
- Active upper gastrointestinal bleeding.
- Recent cardiac arrest <24 hours requiring resuscitation.
- Endotrachial intubation or extubation within 4 hours.

TPN

- 95 to 110 kcal/kg/day.
- 2.2 to 3.5 g protein/kg/day.

16.1   Congenital Heart Disease

Christine Avgeris

16.1.1   Name of Disorder

Congenital heart disease.

16.1.2   Clinical Definition

See the nearby table.

Congenital Heart Disease	
Acyanotic Pressure on left side of heart is greater than right side. Left-to-right shunting causes overcirculation of lungs and may result in congestive heart failure • Atrial septal defect (ASD) • Ventricular septal defect (VSD) • Patent ductus arteriosus (PDA) • Complete atrioventricular canal (CAVC) • Coarctation of aorta • Aortic stenosis	Cyanotic Result of blood flow obstruction of right side of heart Right-to-left shunt results in cyanosis • Tetralogy of Fallot (TOF) • Transposition of the great arteries (TGA) • Tricuspid atresia • Pulmonary atresia • Ebstein anomaly • Total anomalous pulmonary venous return (TAPVR) • Hypoplastic left heart syndrome (HLHS)

16.1.3   How It Is Diagnosed

Physical examination, x-ray, echocardiogram, electrocardiogram.

16.1.4   Nutritional Implications

Children with significant heart disease are at risk for growth failure and malnutrition. In cyanotic lesions, weight and height gain are depressed concurrently. In acyanotic lesions, slow weight gain predominates over linear growth failure.

Factors Contributing to Malnutrition in Cardiac Disease	
Increased Energy Requirements • Increased basal metabolic rate, tachypnea, tachycardia • Increased total energy expenditure • Increased demand of cardiac and respiratory muscle	Decreased Energy Intake • Early satiety or anorexia • Gastroesophageal reflux • Dysphasia

16.1.5   Pearls

- Infants requiring staged repairs such as those with hypoplastic left heart syndrome are at risk for growth failure between repairs. Close monitoring of growth and feeding is important.
- Incidence of growth failure is highest in patients with ventricular septal defect; may be due to greater prevalence of pulmonary hypertension and congestive heart failure.
- Patients who undergo Fontan procedure are at risk for developing protein-losing enteropathy. If this should develop, a high-protein diet low in long-chain fatty acids is usually required. A formula with medium-chain triglycerides (MCTs) is preferred because MCTs are absorbed directly into the portal vein and may be better tolerated.
- Cardiomyopathy is an associated symptom of some metabolic disorders, and nutritional deficiencies such as thiamine, carnitine, or selenium may be present. Trials of thiamine, coenzyme Q, and vitamin C have been used empirically to treat mitochondrial disorders.

Chapter 17

Rheumatology

Nutritional Algorithm for Rheumatic Disease

Rheumatic Disease

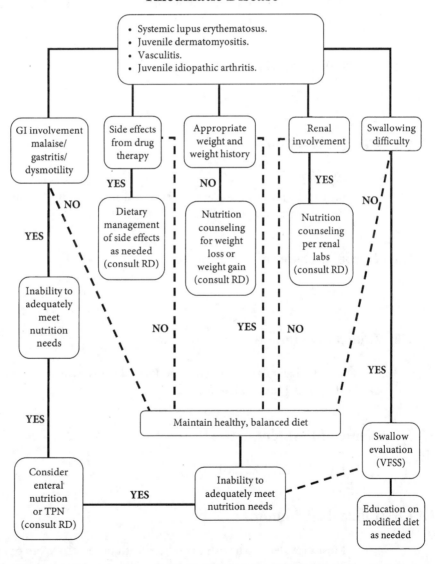

Pediatric Nutrition Handbook: An Algorithmic Approach, First Edition. Edited by David L. Suskind and Polly Lenssen.
© 2011 Blackwell Publishing Ltd. Published 2011 by Blackwell Publishing Ltd.

17.1 Rheumatic Disease
Kim Kellogg

17.1.1 Name of Disorder

Systemic lupus erythematosus (SLE).

17.1.2 Clinical Definition

Characterized by a marked production of autoantibodies, SLE usually affects the connective tissues but can involve multiple organ systems, including kidneys, joints, skin, and blood.

17.1.3 Name of Disorder

Juvenile dermatomyositis (JDMS).

17.1.4 Clinical Definition

Characterized by vasculitis under the skin and in the muscles, resulting in skin rash and gradual muscle weakness and fatigue; also frequently involves skin, lungs, heart, joints, and gastrointestinal (GI) tract.

17.1.5 Name of Disorder

Vasculitis.

17.1.6 Clinical Definition

Destructive inflammation in blood vessel walls, which can result in dysfunction of multiple organ systems.

17.1.7 Name of Disorder

Juvenile idiopathic arthritis (JIA).

17.1.8 Clinical Definition

Most prevalent arthritis in children, with onset <16 years of age, characterized by inflammation, pain, stiffness, swelling, warmth, and/or damage/deformity of joints; can also cause altered bone growth.

17.1.9   Nutrition Implications

- Chronic inflammation can result in muscle atrophy, fatigue, weakness, and significant loss of appetite. Muscle wasting may be replaced with fat, masking a change in body composition.
- Patients are at risk for osteopenia and osteoporosis as a result of inadequate nutrition, chronic inflammation, decreased physical activity, decreased sun exposure, and medication. Adequate vitamin D, calcium intake, and weight-bearing physical activity (as tolerated) reduce the risk for bone loss.
- Patients are at risk for micronutrient deficiencies. Supplementation with a multivitamin is advised.
- Anemia of chronic disease is often present and may coexist with anemia due to iron deficiency or anemia as a side effect of medications. Controlling the underlying disease usually corrects the anemia of chronic disease. Iron supplementation may be necessary.
- Replacement of muscle with fat, a reduction in physical activity, systemic inflammation, and the common use of corticosteroid medications increase risk of premature cardiovascular disease, especially within the SLE population.
- Growth delay can occur as a result of chronic steroid use, increased energy expenditure, and inadequate nutrition. Patients with JIA can experience early epiphyseal fusion.
- Albumin is often decreased because of inflammation and wasting rather than low dietary intake of protein.
- During severe flares of systemic disease or for management of life-threatening macrophage activation syndrome, total parenteral nutrition may be indicated.
- Patients with SLE typically present with a history of anorexia and weight loss.
- Swallowing difficulty and regurgitation can occur due to muscle inflammation and weakness in the throat and esophagus in JDMS. Arthritis in the temporomandibular joint develops in approximately 25% of children with JIA, making chewing and swallowing difficult.

17.1.10   Pearls

- Educating patients and parents about healthy nutrition habits, ensuring adequate nutrient intake, and monitoring growth parameters are the essential aspects of nutrition management in rheumatic disease.
- Assess for symptoms that influence intake and increase risk of malnutrition, such as anorexia, taste changes, problems chewing or swallowing, nausea, pain, vomiting, diarrhea, and signs of poor wound healing.
- Attention should be paid to pain and its effect on food intake.
- If appropriate, exercise is important to the overall health and well-being of these patients.

17.1.11 Nutrition Implications Associated with Drug Therapy

Chronic Glucocorticoid Treatment

- Corticosteroids are commonly used and can result in truncal obesity, decreased muscle mass, decreased bone density, sodium and fluid retention, hypertension, hyperglycemia, increased lipid levels, and increased appetite resulting in weight gain.
- Dietary counseling is often necessary for management of these issues. Calcium and vitamin D supplementation, adequate protein intake, and regular physical activity help mitigate bone loss. A low-sodium diet is indicated to help prevent fluid retention.
- Dietary counseling may be necessary in the setting of weight gain, elevated blood sugar, and elevated lipid levels, as a result of corticosteroid therapy.

Other Side Effects of Drug Therapy

- Immunosuppressive medications can cause GI and liver toxicity and are associated with anorexia, nausea, diarrhea, vomiting, and altered taste, as well as calcium deficiency.
- Methotrexate is associated with folate deficienty and can cause oral ulcers. Standard folic acid supplementation at 1 mg daily minimizes the evolution of oral ulcers.
- Nonsteroidal anti-inflammatory drugs (NSAIDs) are associated with increased risk for folate and iron deficiency. NSAIDs may also cause nausea, vomiting, constipation, gastritis, and GI ulcerations. NSAIDs should be administered after meals.

References

Arthritis Foundation. *Arthritis in Chidren*. Atlanta, GA: Arthritis Foundation, 2009.

Arthritis Foundation. *Nutrition and Your Arthritis*. Atlanta, GA: Arthritis Foundation, 2009.

Coleman, LA. *Nutrition and Rheumatic Disease*. Totowa, NJ: Humana Press; 2008.

Glossary of Acronyms

AA	amino acid; arm area
AAP	American Academy of Pediatrics
AC	arm circumference
AFA	arm fat area
AGE	acute gastroenteritis
ALT	alanine transaminase
AMA	arm muscle area
ARG	arginase deficiency
ARNP	advanced registered nurse practitioner
ASD	atrial septal defect
ASL	argininosuccinate lyase deficiency
ASS	argininosuccinate synthetase deficiency
AST	aspartate transaminase
ATP	adenosine–5′–triphosphate
BCAA	branched-chain amino acids
BEE	basal energy expenditure
BF	breast-feeding
BG	blood glucose
BID	*bis in die* (Latin for "twice daily")
BM	breast milk
BMI	body mass index
BMR	basal metabolic rate
BPD	bronchopulmonary dysplasia
BUN	blood urea nitrogen
Ca	calcium
CACT	carnitine acylcarnitine translocase deficiency
CAVC	complete atrioventricular canal

Pediatric Nutrition Handbook: An Algorithmic Approach, First Edition. Edited by David L. Suskind and Polly Lenssen.
© 2011 Blackwell Publishing Ltd. Published 2011 by Blackwell Publishing Ltd.

CBC	complete blood count
cc	cubic centimeter
CDC	Centers for Disease Control and Prevention
CF	cystic fibrosis
CHD	congenital heart disease
CHO	carbohydrate
CICU	Cardiac Intensive Care Unit
CKD	chronic kidney disease
CLD	chronic lung disease
CMP	cow milk protein allergy
CNS	central nervous system
CPS	carbamyl phosphate synthetase deficiency
CPT 1	carnitine palmitoyl transferase 1 deficiency
CPT 2	carnitine palmitoyl transferase 2 deficiency
CRP	C-reactive protein
CSF	cerebral spinal fluid
D5	dextrose 5%
DASH	Dietary Approaches to Stop Hypertension (diet)
dL	deciliter
DRI	Daily Reference Intake
EAA	essential amino acid
EBM	expressed breast milk
ECLS	extracorporeal life support
ECMO	extracorporeal membrane oxygenation
EER	estimated energy requirement
EFD	estimated fluid deficit
EKG	electrocardiogram
ESRD	end-stage renal disease
FAOD	fatty acid oxidation disorder
FIL	feedback inhibitor of lactation
FTT	failure to thrive
g	gram
GA	gestational age
GA-1	glutaric acidemia type-1
GALT	galactose-1-phosphate uridyltransferase
Gal-1-P	galactose-1-phosphate
GERD	gastroesophageal reflux disease
GFR	glomerular filtration rate
GI	gastroenterology
GSD	glycogen storage disease
Hct	hematocrit
HD	hemodialysis

HFI	hereditary fructose intolerance
Hgb	hemoglobin
HLHS	hypoplastic left heart syndrome
HMF	human milk fortifier
HSCT	hematopoietic stem cell transplantation
HTN	hypertension
IBW	ideal body weight
ICU	intensive care unit
IgA	immunoglobulin A
IgE	immunoglobulin E
IL	intralipid
ILE	isoleucine
IRT	immunoreactive trypsinogen
IU	International Unit
IV	intravenous
IVA	isovaleric acidemia
IVF	intravenous fluid
JDMS	juvenile dermatomyositis
JIA	juvenile idiopathic arthritis
K+	potassium
kcal	kilocalorie
KD	ketogenic diet
kg	kilogram
L	liter
LCHADD	long-chain 3-hydroxy-acyl-CoA dehydrogenase deficiency
LEU	leucine
LFT	liver function test
LYS	lysine
MCADD	medium-chain acyl-CoA dehydrogenase deficiency
MCT	medium-chain triglycerides
mEq	milliequivalent
MET	methionine
mg	milligrams
Mg	magnesium
MI	Motivational Interviewing
mL	milliliter
mm	millimeter
MMA	methylmalonic acidemia
Mmol	millimole
Mmol/L	millimoles/liter
mOsm	milliosmole
mOsm/L	milliosmole/liter

MR	magnetic resonance
MRI	magnetic resonance imaging
MSUD	maple syrup urine disease
MVI	multivitamin
MYCN	V-myc myelocytomatosis viral related oncogene, neuroblastoma derived (avian)

Na+	sodium
NAGS	N-acetylglutamate synthase deficiency
ND	nasoduodenal
ND tube	nasoduodenal tube
NEC	necrotizing enterocolitis
NG	nasogastric
NG tube	nasogastric tube
NICU	neonatal intensive care unit
NPO	*nil per os* (Latin for "nothing per mouth")
NS	normal saline
NSAIDs	nonsteroidal anti-inflammatory drugs

OTC	ornithine transcarbamylase deficiency
OTC	over the counter
OR	operating room
ORS	oral rehydration solution
OT/PT	occupational therapy/physical therapy

PA	propionic acidemia
PAA	plasma amino acid
PCOS	polycystic ovarian syndrome
PDA	patent ductus arteriosus
PGT	per gastrostomy tube
PICU	pediatric intensive care unit
PKU	serum phenylalanine
PN	parenteral nutrition
PO	*per os* (Latin for "by mouth" or orally)
PO_4	phosphate
PPN	peripheral parenteral nutrition
PRN	*pro re nata* (Latin for "as needed")
PTH	parathyroid hormone

RAST	radioallergosorbent test
RBP	retinol-binding protein
RD	registered dietitian
RDA	Recommended Daily Allowance
RDI	Recommended Daily Intake
RMS	rhabdomyosarcoma
R/O	rule out

SAAG	serum ascites-albumin gradient
SLE	systemic lupus erythematosus
SLP	speech-language pathologist
SNS	supplemental nursing system
SSI	Supplemental Security Income
TAPVR	total anomalous pulmonary venous return
Tbsp	tablespoon
TFP	trifunctional protein deficiency
TG	triglycerides
TGA	transposition of the great arteries
THR	threonine
TIBC	total iron-binding capacity
TLC	Therapeutic Lifestyle Changes (diet)
TOF	Tetralogy of Fallot
TPN	total parenteral nutrition
TRP	tryptophan
TSF	triceps skin fold
tsp	teaspoon
tTG	tissue transglutaminase
UA	urinalysis
UCD	urea cycle defects
μg	microgram
UL	upper limit
VAL	valine
VFSS	videofluoroscopic swallow study
VLBW	very low birth weight
VLCADD	very-long-chain acyl-CoA dehydrogenase deficiency
VSD	ventricular septal defect
WHO	World Health Organization
WIC	Women, Infants and Children (Nutritional Program)

Index

Note: Italicized page locators indicate figures; tables are noted with a *t*.